HEAL YOUR
RELATIONSHIP
WITH FOOD

beyoutiful

MARTHA KERR VANCAMP

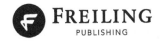

FREILING
PUBLISHING

Published by Freiling Publishing, a division of Freiling Agency, LLC.

P.O. Box 1264,
Warrenton, VA 20188

www.FreilingPublishing.com

ISBN 978-1-950948-63-5

Printed in the United States of America

Dedication

To my patient and amazing husband, Stephen VanCamp. You breathed life into me, you have loved me at every size, and you always remind me that I am beautiful.

To my incredible world-changing children, Sarah, Ian, and Carter.

And to my father and mother, Tom and Lynn Kerr.

Acknowledgments

I'd like to thank my entire #beMarthaFit staff for stepping up and taking on even more as I focused my attention on writing beYOUtiful. Wendy, Jessica, Beth, Liane, Lindsay, Casey, Traci, and Amy, I cannot thank you enough for stepping in the gap.

To my faithful followers and amazing clients, thank you for being my cheerleaders!

Thank you to my publisher, Freiling Publishing, who believed in me and my story and gave me the amazing vehicle to finally tell my story and help thousands more.

Many thanks to my amazing photographer, who is always ready at a moment's notice to shoot all my marketing images. Greg and Chrissy Walck, thank you so much for being on this journey with me.

Additionally, a big thank you to Emily Benko for styling assistance, Haden Reid Boutique, Hotel Haya, and BKN Creative.

Table of Contents

Preface

I have lived my life and weight-loss journey very openly for the last nine years. I've always said that I'm an open book, through which I have assisted and cared for thousands throughout their journey. But all this comes with haters and people who mock me for living my life out loud. I just don't care. My mess is my message, and I'd be remiss if I lived my life any other way. Through my mess, I found my beYOUtiful purpose. And I subscribe to the belief that our mission in life is to discover our purpose and then give it away.

Never be afraid of your mess. Never be afraid of living your life out loud. You have no idea the positive, powerful impact you can have on one or thousands of others just for owning your mess and turning it into your message.

Remember: Your story has power, and it can help you and others heal together.

Are you ready? You are about to embark on a life-altering journey that will uncover the most beYOUtiful version of you and finally heal your relationship with food. When you're done, I will be excited to hear all about it.

A quick note for you: As you read the book, don't stop after section 2 and start your journey. Section 3 is vitally important to the long-term success of your journey.

Section 1

Chapter 1

The Doctor's Visit That Changed My Life

Morbidly Obese!

I read those two damning words on my chart!

I literally wanted to vomit.

I was forty years old, on my second marriage, and raising seven children while my husband was deployed.

I was undone. I was working full time and was barely surviving the load that comes with being a single parent of seven. My dinners consisted of a bottle of wine followed by sleeping pills.

The doctor's visit was merely routine to check my thyroid, which I had "blown out" due to an estrogen overload when I was pregnant with my twins, twelve years prior. As I left the office with my personal printout folded over so I couldn't see my weight from the visit, a fateful wind (literally) blew the paper from my hands and revealed the ugly truth.

I weighed well over 250 pounds and now had the label of "morbidly obese"!

This was a life-changing day that presented a series of opportunities. These opportunities I chose to act upon, and in doing so, I dramatically altered the course of not only my life, but also thousands of other lives across the world.

This is my story, my reality, and the story of how I hit rock bottom and rebuilt victoriously. I dropped from 250+ pounds to 142 pounds, and I am now at a very healthy maintenance weight. I will guide you to heal your relationship with food. I will walk you through the exact steps you need to make the mindset shift, to create your sustainable plan, and the most important part—to walk your imperfect journey. Additionally, I will provide you with resources, sustainable weight-loss meal plans, and recipes.

You should approach this book as a living roadmap or blueprint to success. You will want to read it thoroughly and return often. I have separated the book into sections for ease of use. But plan on reading this from beginning to end, at first.

At some point in life, most people will utter the words: "I want to lose weight!"

As a master wellness and weight loss coach, I will tell you what everyone really wants: confidence, self-assurance, self-love, and less anxiety and depression. Losing weight is a means to an end, and therefore I say: Fix Your Food, Fix Your Life.

Chapter 2

Your Line in the Sand

Big or small, everyone has a defining moment. You draw a line in the sand and say NO MORE.

I mentioned my moment: the parking lot of the doctor's office, the fateful wind that literally blew open the folded paper that listed my weight, blood pressures, and all the vitals.

When that wind blew the paper from my hands and it landed wide open inside my car, on the passenger seat, curiosity killed the cat.

I wanted to see the information, but at the same time, I didn't. I was scared.

I looked anyway.

I saw my blood pressure: low.

I saw my height: 6 feet.

I saw my weight: 265 pounds.

But it was the next two words that made me crumble: Morbidly Obese.

What? What happened to me? I now had a label: Morbidly Obese. Now I was more than a number defined by the scale—I had a label.

For me the word "obese" is horrible. But the added word "MORBIDLY" shook me up.

It wasn't that very day that I drew my line in the sand. It would be a few months more.

In May of that same year, for one entire week, I awoke and heard a voice in the back of my head. For three mornings, it was the same voice and the same question: "What are you going to do now, Martha?"

On the fourth day, the voice got louder and more urgent: "Martha! What are you going to do now?!"

It was five days, the same voice, and the same general question. But the last two days were strong and authoritative.

I knew this was my window of opportunity to fix me. I knew without a doubt that I had to immediately walk my journey. No one could help me. No one was coming to save me. This was up to me. I can honestly say, looking back, if I hadn't acted right then, I never would have, and I'd be living a very destructive life right now.

May 2012 was my line in the sand.

You have either had or are about to have that moment—you'll hear that "voice" in the back of our head. Call it the Holy Spirit, call it the Universe, or call it your intuition. We all have a guiding light in our lives, and it generally shows up as a tiny voice that can get louder and more insistent. It's your choice whether you listen and learn from it.

NEVER IGNORE THIS VOICE.

NEVER IGNORE A WINDOW OF OPPORTUNITY.

WALK BY FAITH TO AND THROUGH THIS OPPORTUNITY.

For decades, I trusted everyone else with my weight issue. I knew this time that it was up to me to educate myself and to learn what and when to eat. I became my first client. Within the first ten months, I had lost 50+ pounds. I saw the number 200 on the scale, and I was thrilled. I thought I was done.

I felt incredible. I was confident. I was wearing a size 14 and elated to be out of a size 22 and 2XL.

It felt incredible to purge my closet. I had started my journey at the beginning of the summer, and by fall, I literally had no clothes that fit me. By winter, I was buying a whole new wardrobe. The following summer, I had to start all over with every piece of clothing.

I would purge, give clothes to my neighbors, and donate the rest. I vividly remember a few of my neighbors commenting that they felt I was giving away my clothes too soon. What they were implying was, surely, I would be gaining the weight back, like every other person does. But I knew I was never going back. I may stumble, but I was never going back to my starting weight. Ever.

Over the next several years, my pattern was the same: lose, maintain, and then lose some more.

By 2016, I hit my all-time low: 142 pounds. This was too skinny, but we'll talk later about the race for skinny versus healthy.

Have you drawn your line in the sand? Great. You are at a state of readiness. Now it's time to walk TO and THROUGH the opportunity in front of you.

Or are you waiting to hear the voice that will prompt you to start your journey? If this is the case, sweet friend, allow your decision to buy this book to be your sign to draw that line and start your journey!

Don't overthink; there is never the "right" or "perfect" time to start. Just start.

Chapter 3

The Beginning of Your Journey

Losing weight is on the list as one of the most difficult and emotional projects you will endure. I know—I've lived it!

Losing ten or twenty pounds often involves the same emotional process as having to lose over one hundred pounds. The process is the same, and the feelings are the same. No matter what, there is never a shortcut.

When some women run to #beMarthaFit, I look at their pictures and think, "Why do they think they need or want to lose weight?" What I've come to realize, after nearly a decade of coaching, is no matter the size or weight, clients all want the same thing: to feel confident, to love themselves, to feel energetic, and able to conquer their days with ease. To achieve all this, it always comes down to one thing: FOOD! So if you have only ten or fifteen pounds to lose, rock on, friend—I get it. And while you may not have the emotional baggage that often comes with a decade(s)-long weight issue, your needs and desires are just as important, and you will want to work through sections 2 and 3 of this book.

Always remember that your mindset will determine your success. You already know this, but remember, nothing will change unless you choose to change!

To put it simply: You will never change your life until you change something you do daily. Every single day!

None of us are accustomed to putting ourselves on the daily TO-DO list. No one is continuously strong enough to say "no" to trigger foods or to heavy-drinking social events. And women, listen up, you are wired to put everyone (kids, husband, significant other, even your job) first, before your own health and well-being. Doing this has likely come at your own expense.

It will not be an easy task to unlearn habits or even to say "no" to others, including family. But this is the task at hand. As I said, nothing will change unless you decide to change your priorities and your social events, and to put yourself on the daily TO-DO list.

You have an opportunity staring you in the face. You have a chance to walk with me and heal your relationship with food. But your mindset must be strong, and you have to be willing to drop your list of excuses and commit to putting yourself first.

So let's do it!

As you work through this book, I want you to know that I have lived this, and I'm honored to now guide you through an amazing, wonderful, incredible, and freeing journey. But only you can do the work. No one is going to do it for you. No one is coming to save you. YOU oversee your progress, and as you progress, you will hit obstacles. The journey is never perfect. However, when you do hit obstacles, I want you to continually assess this: Where are you on the daily TO-DO list?

Chapter 4

Who Do You Love

I coach busy moms, career women, and women in their twenties all the way to grandmas. No matter the age, there is always a common theme of putting everyone else first and gladly, willingly not caring about their own bodies. I was guilty of this as well for decades!

One of the biggest issues I continually see with women is their innate ability to put themselves last. I have so many women clients who would rather "hide" behind taking care of their husbands, kids, and careers rather than putting their own health first. I call this "willingly sitting in a destructive hole."

Time after time, day after day, I coach women who tell me they clearly know their own physical and mental health is rapidly going downhill. They start my program, only to fall on their face within the first twelve weeks. And no amount of my coaching can help them because they continually go back to sitting in a destructive hole, by choice! I can't pull them out—no one can pull them out. They must choose not to return to the destructive hole.

So what happens in this hole? NOTHING GOOD. Nothing happens that will promote your health, ease your anxiety, or lead to sustainable, long-term weight loss. But rather, in this destructive hole, as you spend your time caring for everyone else or striving for a new job title or more money, you will be saying YES to everyone but yourself. Nowhere in this destructive hole is time for you! Everyone and everything else always win, and you end up another day, month, or year in the same spot (or worse) health-wise.

Scarily, a lot of women would rather stay in this destructive hole than to do the work that needs to be done, and to say "no" to others, in order to put their health first.

So, here's our first exercise. Buckle up!

You ready?

Get out a piece of paper and pen.

Now…

List the five people you love the most.

Now review your list.

Are YOU even on the list?

The first time I made this list, I shocked myself. It was 2016, well into my wellness journey, and I was married to my second husband (my forever husband) Stephen.

Here was my list of the five people I love the most:

1. God

2. My husband, Stephen

3. My three children

4. My mother

5. My best friend, Lesley

I reviewed my list and followed the next instruction: Am I even on the list?

I laughed. NOPE!

When I took this test, it was toward the end of my weight-loss journey. It was wildly eye-opening, and I wish I had taken this "test" early on.

This simple test will help you throughout your journey, reminding you that the joyful sacrifice you are making to put YOUR own health as a priority is vitally important. You will continually have to reassess the top five people you love and remind yourself to put YOU on that list.

For women, especially, you won't put yourself on the list. You don't even think twice about it. You list everyone else. You list the people you care for. But the thought of caring for yourself is so foreign. Or you have bought into what the world tells you: Caring for yourself is selfish.

And therein lies the first problem.

Think of it this way: The airplane is going down. What do the flight attendants tell you to do? Put the oxygen mask on yourself before helping others (including your children).

Self-love, taking care of yourself, making your health a priority, is far from selfish. Many of my clients come to me in their forties. I find that somewhere in their forties, women tend to "wake up." They realize their children are old enough to be somewhat independent, their careers (if they have one outside of the home) are blossoming, and they have had days or weeks when they realize they have "lost themselves" taking care of everyone and everything else in their lives.

I love working with these clients if they realize it's their job to pull themselves out of the destructive hole. No coach can do that for them. And even when these women draw their own line in the sand and begin to take back their lives and their own health, it's a daily challenge to stay out of the destructive hole.

Remember, you allowed your children, your spouse, your job, or your aging parents to put you in the destructive hole. You've been busy doing life for everyone else. YOU ALLOWED THIS. So every day, you're going to have to be proactive and not allow these same people and circumstances to push you back down into the hole. **It's your choice.**

For some, the hole of destruction is a comfort zone. As yucky as it feels, the anxiety that comes with it, the self-loathing feelings you have each day, oddly enough, that hole can feel like a comfort zone. But you know the saying: Nothing good comes from remaining in your comfort zone.

Chapter 5

Doing This For You

I married my first husband at age twenty-four. He was the first Christian man I dated after graduating with a BFA in electronic media from the University of Cincinnati. My sisters, Deb (ten years older) and Cathy (seven years older), married their college sweethearts, both Christians, after graduating from a small private Christian college in western Pennsylvania. I figured if they married their college sweethearts, and if the man I was dating was a Christian, then this man must be the man I'm supposed to marry.

Early on, prior to be being engaged, I knew my now ex-husband had his own confidence issues. He made it known at certain times that he didn't like his own weight, and rightfully so. At this point in my life, I weighed just over 200 pounds and wore a size 14. I quietly had my own dislike for my weight, but it wasn't affecting me daily. I didn't necessarily feel fat or ugly. I was in a good headspace. My future husband wasn't.

We were engaged, and soon after we set our wedding for October 12, 1996, we began premarital counseling with the pastor who would marry us. Each week, we were given homework assignments that we were expected to complete. Most of these assignments were benign.

Until this one...

Tell each other something that bothers you now that you fear could become an issue later in life.

This was easy for me to answer, and I knew what I had to say wouldn't cut him to his core: "I don't like the way you procrastinate and take forever to finish or complete things."

That was easy enough. It was truth, and I had already experienced his inability to complete tasks that didn't necessarily have a set deadline. It bothered me, and it was something we had talked about before.

Then he said the following, and it's a direct quote, because I will never ever forget these words. They are burnt into my brain and I will take them to my grave.

He said, "I'm worried our children will be embarrassed by you; I don't want them growing up with a fat mom!"

I thought to myself: I AM NOT FAT!

My hands still shake every time I tell this story, as they are right now. That one sentence paralyzes me every time I think, speak, or write it.

I remember exactly where I was in my apartment when he said this. We both were lying in my bed. I had no idea this bomb was going to be lobbed my way. There was no warning. I was blindsided.

"I'm worried our children will be embarrassed by you; I don't want them growing up with a fat mom!"

I immediately began to cry quietly. It was dark, and I was thankful that he couldn't see the tears streaming down my face. I slowly asked my first question, my voice low and quiet, while trying so hard not to reveal the tears: "Why? Why would you say that?"

He stumbled to answer. He was struggling to put sentences together. But he made it known that I wasn't at an OK weight for him. I didn't have the body that he envisioned for his soon-to-be wife. And he followed up by saying: "I was embarrassed by my mom growing up. I didn't like that she was so overweight."

It would take over a decade for me to realize that my future husband was projecting his own insecurities on me, that his comment truly had NOTHING to do with me, but rather his own issue with his weight and his mother's weight.

I'm a people-pleaser. And, to this day, I still struggle with continually striving for an unrealistic level of perfection. At that time, I desperately wanted to please him and to be accepted and loved for my body.

In the following weeks, I began exercising (which I hated), and I immediately saw a doctor and begged for diet pills. I got them. I wanted to please my future husband. I wanted him to love me and to think I was beautiful. I was doing all of this for HIM—NOT for me.

On the day we married, I weighed 194 pounds. I looked gorgeous in my wedding dress. I felt beautiful, and my father told me I looked "stunning." It was a perfect day. I had lost weight for my husband, and all I wanted to hear from him was "You are beautiful."

In my entire marriage, I never heard those words. Never.

I was married to a man who, at his core, had so many insecurities that he had no ability to love me. He certainly never complimented me or showed me that I was beautiful in his eyes. In fact, years later, his words about my body became extremely destructive, which ultimately was the demise of our marriage.

All the diets I tried and failed at during my marriage to my first husband were, at the very core, to please him, to have him notice me, and to be acknowledged. I never did it for me. So, of course, I failed. Doing it to please him meant when times got tough, or I hit a plateau, I didn't want it badly enough to push on and continue. Nor was I getting any affirmation of the effort I was making. So why would I do it?

So let me ask you: Are you doing this for you?

Or are you doing this because a mother, a sister, a husband, or a boyfriend wants you to be skinnier? If the answer to this question is YES, put the book down. Now is not YOUR time. **If you try to execute the #beMarthaFit way now, you will fail.**

I can't help you. No one can help you unless you want this for YOU.

Remember, no one is coming to save you. No one is going to do this for you. You must want it badly. Your desire for change must be so infectious that no matter what comes your way, you won't quit.

Right now, you are going into a battle that you can and will win. But you must go into battle with yourself and with your body, and a NO-FAIL attitude is expected.

Will you fall along the way? Sure.

Will you have bad days? Of course.

Will you question WHY you started? You sure will.

Will you win every battle? No.

But is it worth it? Without a doubt.

And YOU WILL WIN THE WAR.

And so, you must do this FOR YOU and no one else. Because, my dear friend, if you do this the right way, you will learn that by simply fixing your food, you will fix your life.

Right now, make sure YOU want this. You want this for you and no one else.

Chapter 6

The Secret Sauce

In 2009, my divorce to my first husband was finalized. Later that year, I married Stephen. Fast forward to 2016, I achieved nearly a 105-pound loss, and I realized so much in my life had changed and evolved for good.

My second marriage to Stephen was thriving.

My business was thriving.

I had never genuinely felt happier, stronger, or confident.

I felt unstoppable.

Nothing that came my way rocked me.

I felt light.

My brain felt clear.

For the first time ever, I felt that I was leading the most authentic life. I felt like the "real" Martha had been uncovered.

And as a successful weight loss and wellness coach, at that time, I wanted to dive deeply and figure out WHY everything in my life was lining up and why I felt that I was operating on a high-performance level.

I wanted to bottle this feeling and offer it to my clients and friends.

I realized after a short time of self-analysis and discovery that I didn't need to bottle this.

Everyone already had IT.

So, what is IT?

FOOD!

Now, don't blow me off, skip this chapter, or even roll your eyes at me.

The way I was feeling, the way I was operating, I credit to the food I was eating and had been eating, consistently, for the previous four years. No joke!

Let's talk science for just a moment. Let's explore the gut-to-brain connection.

At the very simplest level, the gut connects with the brain through chemicals, including hormones, as well as neurotransmitters that send messages. A troubled gut can send messages to the brain and the brain to the gut. These messages include anxiety, stress, and depression. All of this is transmitted through the nerves in your body.

It's as if these two vital organs are talking to each other. The good, the bad, and the ugly are discussed.

Now think about this: What passes through your gut?

FOOD!

Food passes from the stomach through a tube that leads to the intestines and then through another tube before going to the colon. It's the small intestines that absorb nutrients and the liquids from the foods you eat and drink.

Your small intestines (part of your gut) take a beating! It's likely taken a beating for years, even decades. For me, it was a thirty-year beating.

Refined sugar, skipped meals, lack of sleep and/or recovery, overeating, processed foods, lack of water, stress, and more all affect the health of your gut.

But step back and look at that list again.

What CAN YOU CONTROL on that list?

I'll tell you.

The answer is: What you put in your mouth!

FOOD!

What I thought was special, how I was feeling and operating, wasn't special at all.

I was feeling this way because of the whole foods, nutrient-dense foods, and predominantly single ingredient foods I was eating.

There's truly nothing magical about it.

But it quickly became evident that what I was offering to my clients was working magic in their lives.

My clients were fixing their food and fixing their lives.

Clients were experiencing life without anxiety and depression.

Clients were reducing their dependence on pills.

Clients were discovering they had the strength to exit abusive relationships.

Clients had the confidence to ask for the promotion at work and get it.

Clients had the confidence to go back to school and start new careers that they wanted for years.

Clients felt strong enough to tackle their breaking marriages and save them.

I have watched thousands of clients each year either take back control over their lives or pave new thriving paths for their lives.

You have this same power. But it will start with fixing your food. For when you fix your food, you will heal from the inside out. You will create a healthy gut, and in turn, that healthy gut will send beautiful messages to your brain.

What you eat is your ticket to a changed life.

Don't believe me? Try this: Eat all the processed foods and alcohol you want for two or three days. Then assess how you feel!

Are you proud of yourself?

Do you feel confident?

Do you have the strength to tackle pressing issues?

Are you performing at a high level at work?

Are you being patient with your children or spouse?

Every time I personally choose to "loosen the reigns" on my food plan and eat off-plan and drink alcohol, I lose a day or more to negative emotions. I lose my footing. I don't feel confident to lead. I'm in no shape to coach. And I spin. ONE day of eating wildly off-plan, and I'm messy. I hate myself. And I pile on the guilt trip.

Back to your crazy experiment: after two or three days of a food and alcohol binge, start eating whole foods, single-ingredient foods, and nutrient-dense foods. In as short as a day or two, you will awake with energy, a positive mind, a happy heart, a spring in your step, and confidence. Negative thoughts will quiet. You'll be calmer, more patient.

You will begin to LOVE you. And when you LOVE YOU, you're unstoppable.

It's not magic.

It's food.

When you eat predominantly processed foods, with ingredients you cannot pronounce, or when alcohol (poison) is a daily or weekly part of your life, you are asking your gut to digest, metabolize, and function with food that truly ISN'T food—it's chemicals. And your body doesn't know how to digest those chemicals. So, it sits there, ferments, and increases gut inflammation.

This will quickly lead to bigger issues that you will physically feel:

Chronic constipation.

Mood disorders.

Irritable bowel syndrome.

Asthma.

Diabetes.

The list goes on and on.

And even now, Harvard Health has published an entire article on how scientists are learning more and more about how the trillions of bacteria dwelling deep inside your digestive tract can affect your risk of cardiovascular disease.

It's time to really approach what you want for your life and what you're eating. The magic is right in front you.

Food.

Fix your food, and you'll fix your life.

Chapter 7

What is Food

I was nine years old and remember starting my first diet. The game plan was to eat 1,200 calories or less. Just do that, and losing weight would be simple. For me? Not so much. I'd lose a little, but I felt like I was starving, and truthfully, I was.

The yo-yo diet cycle was very real for me. Binge eating. Dieting. Shame. Guilt. Self-loathing. This was my reality for 30+years.

Diet pills.

Laxatives.

Juicing.

Nutrisystem.

Weight Watchers.

Prepackaged weight-loss foods.

The Diet Coke and Cheez-Its diet. What? You haven't heard of that one? I created this diet, and honestly, this was my plan for several months.

All of these were my plans. My plans to get me to "skinny"!

When I was in college, my father gave me a credit card for emergencies. I used it to pay for a lifetime membership to Nutrisystem. He wasn't thrilled when I called to tell him the news.

My best (and most expensive) weight loss plan was to cut it all off—plastic surgery for the win. I started this in my early thirties. To date, I've had the following surgeries:

>   Thigh lift
>
>   Extended tummy tuck
>
>   Breast reduction and lift
>
>   Arm reduction

The one item I didn't follow through with was gastric bypass.

But guess what? None of MY plans worked, not even plastic surgery! None of them were sustainable. And even after numerous plastic surgeries, I ballooned up to over 250 pounds.

WHY?

Because I never FIXED MY FOOD.

Fixing your food is where we must start, but as you know, that can be overwhelming. So let's immediately break through the clutter, the misinformation on the internet. Let's start by talking about why FOOD IS FUEL.

FOOD IS FUEL.

The easiest visual I can give you is your car. You would never ask your car to run without gas. Food is fuel to your body, like gas is to a car. Your body, on a cellular level, requires food to operate. But your body requires whole foods, nutrient-dense foods, and single-ingredient foods—not the processed, grab-and-go foods you've likely been putting in your body. Think of it his way: your body requires high-octane gas, not the cheap unleaded gas you've been filling up with.

The lack of quality fuel isn't entirely your fault. You've been duped. Food manufacturers are slick at marketing, and they are leading you into believe that what you're eating is healthy, when in fact, it's not.

Let's break down exactly what you need to know. Your body needs key macronutrients. Macronutrients are the building blocks to calories, and they provide the energy you need as well as the repair work your body needs. Macros are the nutrients you cannot live without.

They are:

> Lean protein
>
> Complex carbohydrates
>
> Healthy fats

Each one of these macronutrients serves a purpose in your body functioning properly. In an upcoming chapter, I'll outline what exactly constitutes lean protein, complex carbohydrates, and healthy fats!

Let's start with LEAN PROTEIN. Your body uses protein to build and repair tissues. You also use protein to make enzymes, hormones, and other body chemicals. Protein is an important building block of bones, muscles, cartilage, skin, and blood.

COMPLEX CARBS. This is an energy source for your body—specifically, your muscles. When you eat complex carbs, they turn into glucose (blood sugar), which in turn becomes energy. And glucose is used in the cells of the brain and body.

HEALTHY FATS. This is also an energy source for your body. Fats provide energy to the organs, aid in absorbing nutrients, and produce important hormones. And let's clear up misinformation: Eating fat doesn't make you fat.

In order of importance, you should focus first on protein, and then choose an energy source: complex carbs or healthy fats.

Your body also needs micronutrients (vitamins and minerals), but it's the MACROnutrients that allow your body to function properly.

You'll notice I haven't even mentioned CALORIES. Why? I don't need to, because each one of the above-mentioned macronutrients carries a caloric level. So once we determine what your macrostructure looks like, we will know how many calories you need to maintain, gain, or lose weight. We'll cover building your plan in Section 2 of this book.

Fixing your food is the foundation of weight loss. Not exercise. Not supplements. The foundation is built with food.

You know this: You cannot outrun your fork. No amount of working out or supplementation can create long-standing sustainable results.

In fact, I had a client who started with me named Holly. She was wildly successful with the program, and in nine months, she lost sixty-eight pounds. One of the main reasons Holly chose to become a #beMarthaFit client was because I don't require exercise for fat loss.

Holly looked at me one day and said, "I'm allergic to exercise!"

We still have a great laugh over this comment.

I will prove to you that exercise is not, and never will be, in the "blueprint" for losing weight. Only real food!

The only role exercise will play is in reshaping the physique of your body. You want beautiful, rounded shoulders? Pick up some weights. You want more muscular definition? Work out.

Yes, muscle burns fat. By no means am I disputing this fact. However, I want to make it very clear to you that by simply fixing your food, you will lose weight. Working out is a bonus. Just remember, the foundation to losing weight all starts with your food choices, not your time in the gym.

Chapter 8

Understanding Macros

As a forty-year-old, I remember taking my first nutrition class. I left the class feeling hopeful and yet super overwhelmed. At that point, I knew enough to be dangerous. My next thought was, what now? No one gave me a structured plan. No one gave me calories or macronutrients. So I set out to wing this and determined to trust no one other than myself. I knew I would stumble a lot and fail many days, but I was determined and passionate not to give up on ME: my first client.

So here we are. You are now your own client. You are special, you are amazing, and you are going to finally heal your relationship with food. But I wouldn't blame you if you're overwhelmed. Consider yourself a baby. No one is asking you to roll over or walk at this point. Sit back and be cared for, just as you would care for a newborn.

I tell my clients, let me do the thinking for you, so I'll do the same for you.

So, Coach Martha, what's next?

We'll build your blueprint to success in Section 2 of this book, but let's list some foods within each macronutrient group.

Lean Protein Sources:
Chicken breast
Pork loin
Egg whites
White fish
Turkey breast
Bison
Red meat—fattier
Salmon—fattier
Lamb

Complex Carb Sources:
Rice
Sweet potatoes
Couscous
Quinoa
Black beans

Healthy Fat Sources:
Avocados
Some cheeses
Nuts and seeds
Hummus
Nut butters
Whole eggs
Fattier fishes such as salmon and some cuts of beef

So many times, as a wellness and weight-loss coach, I feel the need to defend carbohydrates. They get a bad rap. It's not the fault of carbs that we associate them as being bad. There is a big difference between fast-releasing carbs and complex carbs.

Throughout elementary school, middle school, and into high school, I was on a 1,200-calorie diet, and I was starving all the time. I would sneak food into the finished basement of our central Pennsylvania home after school. Often it was a box of Lucky Charms, Cinnamon Life cereal, or my all-time favorite, a Pop-Tart—but not just any Pop-Tart. This was the toasted strawberry flavor, and once it was crisp and warm, I would take real butter and pat it on the breaded side of the Pop-Tart. It had that delicious combination of bread, sugary frosting, a warm strawberry middle, and salty butter on top. Talk about heaven in my mouth.

Pop-Tarts are a fast-releasing carb, so this food doesn't have a place in any meal plan. I know—I'm sad about it, too.

Fast-releasing carbs will release glucose into the bloodstream, causing a near-instant spike in your blood sugar. You may feel high and full of energy within sixty seconds. But just as quickly, you will feel a crash, feel "foggy," or even feel a need to nap. Sadly, there is nothing good about this quick UP and DOWN. Fast-releasing carbs will lead to many chronic diseases.

For the most part, there is no need to fully eliminate complex carbs from your lifestyle eating plan. There may be purposeful reasons to periodically go low-carb or remain at a low-carb intake due to some health diagnosis (such as insulin resistance and/or PCOS). But always remember each macronutrient that we have outlined serves a purpose in keeping your body operational.

Together, in Section 2 of this book, I will walk you through calculating calories and macros and building your weight-loss meal plan.

Chapter 9

Why This Works

When I started my weight-loss journey trusting only myself, I approached my journey with blind faith. I had no clue I would end up losing 105 pounds. I suppose I knew in my heart this would be different. It felt right, but absolutely I had blind faith, and in some way, I'm asking you to have the same blind faith.

As you work through this book, I'm sure you're wondering WHY would this journey be any different?

Why will it work this time?

Trust me; you will be wildly successful if you keep these three words in mind: Education, Sustainability, and Sacrifice.

Remember the 1,200-calorie diet I was on (and likely you have been on) for decades? That was, and continues to be, a massive failure. Nearly fifty years ago, scientists declared that women would need to eat approximately 1,200 calories a day to lose weight, and men would need 1,700 calories.

We know now that this "scientific model" was and is ridiculous. But if your mother put you on this caloric restriction, is was no fault of hers. It was all our mothers knew and understood! But we know better now.

If you have trusted what I call "big box" national weight-loss companies and have failed, I get it. I've been down that road with you and failed.

Here are a just few reasons why:

You relied on a point system. All foods are allowed if you count the points. **Why this is flawed:** All calories are not created equal. Not all foods should be allowed, as many of them are not whole foods, nutrient-dense foods, or single-ingredient foods. Additionally, you merely count points. You aren't learning about macronutrients, and you aren't learning the science behind food. Ask yourself: Do you really want to count points for the rest of your life?

You relied on pre-packaged food. This system sets you up for failure from day one. You have no idea why you are eating what you're eating. You have no further education, and do you really want to eat pre-packaged foods for the rest of your life? Additionally, this is very lifestyle-limiting. How are you supposed to navigate social events with success? Eating out becomes a disaster.

I could spend chapters and chapters outlining why I feel so many trusted weight loss systems are failing you. Rather than focusing on the flawed, let's spend our time talking about what works and why it works.

Three words: Education, Sustainability, and Sacrifice.

EDUCATION. You need to understand why certain foods are better than others. You need to understand the science behind how your body reacts and metabolizes food sources. You need to understand macronutrients and nutrition labels.

SUSTAINABILITY. You need to approach your journey as a life-long journey. This is no longer about diets. This is a long-term approach to eating for optimal health and mental wellness. There is no endpoint; there isn't a finish line. So always ask yourself: Is what I'm doing NOW something I know I can execute the rest of my life? The #beMarthaFit way is.

SACRIFICE. This may be the hardest part to comprehend and execute long term. You can't expect any change without joyful sacrifice. That might be sacrifice of time, money, friendships, choices, or behaviors. I use this analogy with my clients. If you want to take the vacation of a lifetime or purchase a Gucci purse, it comes with a sacrifice somewhere in your life. Unless you win the lottery, neither of those wishes will come to fruition without a financial sacrifice somewhere else. The same needs to be applied to your lifestyle eating plan.

Your sacrifices for success will mean that you will take time to prep your food, you will choose to sanitize your environment so you aren't tempted by the crap you have been living off of, you will stop drinking that nightly beer or glass(es) of wine after work, you will stop going through a fast-food drive-thru, and you will stop "being on plan" throughout the week and bingeing on the weekends. You will say NO to girlfriends who get together only to drink. You no longer will celebrate with food; you will pause before you emotionally eat.

YES, there must be a sacrifice—a JOYFUL sacrifice. What are you willing to give up to put YOUR HEALTH on the TO-DO LIST?

If you can agree that you need assistance cutting through the noise on the internet and educate yourself by immersing in this book...

If you can agree that you will no longer diet but rather approach this as a new lifestyle...

If you can agree that you must put yourself on the daily TO-DO list and that you are willing to define the areas you are willing to sacrifice and make room for your health...

THEN YOU WILL BE WILDLY SUCCESSFUL.

Always remember: Education, Sustainability, and a JOYFUL Sacrifice.

Chapter 10

The Joyful Sacrifice

I began my journey to lose weight for the last time at the age of 40. I decided I would not only change the food I was eating, but I would also not have any alcohol for eight weeks! This was my commitment to myself and my body!

Before we begin Section 2 of the book and create your food blueprint to success, I want to remind you once again that all of this comes with a sacrifice. But with sacrifice comes an amazing reward, a payoff of sorts.

Your food blueprint will mean giving up your go-to comfort foods and drinks. Not permanently, but for a period, and then when they are reintroduced, it will be within parameters.

I cannot say this enough: you must make "room" for this new way of eating. There won't be any room for this new lifestyle if you aren't willing to give up in other areas of your life.

Now, I can imagine that many of you are already mourning the events, the foods, and the drinks you will be asked to give up, but listen to me: The last several decades of your life have literally been a treat meal.

For me, the first forty years of my life were my treat meal, except for the times when I was dieting.

I would eat the cake when I wanted the cake.

I would order pizza when I wanted pizza.

I would join friends for margaritas any time they asked.

My life was a treat meal.

Stop mourning the things you are about to give up. Flip the script in your head and begin listing all the WINS you want to experience:

Walking into any store and fitting into everything you try on

Taking fewer medications

Perhaps being able to sit comfortably in a restaurant booth

Maybe sitting on a plane without the seat belt extender

Being able to bend over and tie your own shoes

No longer dreading doctor visits

Being able to walk or run, long distances, without feeling exhausted

Waking up every day without aches and pains

Not having your hands or feet swollen and painful

Not experiencing intestinal distress

Enduring less sickness

Sweet friend, the list is literally endless. And most importantly, you will soon be adding days to the end of your life rather than shortening your life by the foods you are eating.

You've had a lifetime of treat meals. And where did that get you? You may be sad, depressed, and filled with self-loathing, with a closet of clothes that don't fit.

Treat meal is over (although I promise to walk you through how to period-ically enjoy an off-plan meal).

Now, the joyful sacrifice begins.

Section 2

Introduction

Section 2 is all about creating your blueprint to success. I will walk you through, step by step, to determine the caloric and macronutrient numbers you need to crunch and how to fill up your day with the proper fuel.

This section is chock full of so much information that it may cause to you feel overwhelmed. There is a large learning curve in this section as I am consolidating a decade of knowledge and action steps into a few short chapters.

At any moment you feel on overload, stop. Take a break. Remember, no one is asking you to be an expert out of the gate. Always remember, you can reach out to me if you need additional help.

If this process were easy, everyone would do it, and everyone would be wildly successful. But considering over 70 percent of Americans are overweight, this clearly isn't easy. A word of warning: Without consistent support, you may find you have many starts and stops. Support is vitally important, as is accountability. Sadly, when I hand someone a customized meal plan and that person hasn't signed up for support and accountability, there is a very high failure rate. Remember, we weren't built to do hard things alone. However, when we combine a sustainable food plan with support and accountability, there is a 95 percent success rate.

Remember, asking for help isn't a sign of weakness. Many of you have a financial planner or a business coach. These people in your life are experts in their fields, and they guide you to success. The same can be said for hiring a weight-loss coach. In this case, I am your expert, and there is no shame in asking for additional help or turning your journey over to the expert.

Chapter 11

Wellness as Weight Loss

I used to believe that all I had to do was diet, eat less, and my body would respond. To be clear, that's what 100 percent of my clients also believe, until I explain the complexities of wellness.

My goal is to arm you with as much information as possible without bogging down your brain or getting too deeply into science. So let's start here by defining wellness.

The health of your cells, hormones, and organs all dictate your wellness. For the sake of this book, we'll categorize wellness as weight loss. And for this very reason, there will never be a one-size-fits-all approach to weight loss.

There are four contributing factors to wellness/weight loss:

Thyroid health

Hormones

Adrenal glands

Mitochondria

If you have ever consulted your primary care doctor for weight loss, he or she will generally test your thyroid health. Some doctors stop there, leaving you with very little to no answers. And yes, some people may never be treated for hypothyroidism even though they have symptoms, because their thyroid stimulating hormone (TSH) levels are well within normal range.

Some doctors will proceed with hormone testing; however, most will tell you these tests aren't needed if you're getting your period regularly.

Your thyroid health and hormones are massive pieces to the puzzle when it comes to weight loss, but let's go even deeper.

Your adrenal glands sit atop each of your kidneys. These tiny glands are powerful and produce hormones, including sex hormones and cortisol. When you have an issue with your adrenal glands, they either make too much or not enough of the hormones your body needs. Cortisol helps you respond to stress, and when those levels increase excessively, your body can become insulin resistant. That can lead to an increase in blood sugar, weight gain, and potentially type 2 diabetes. When cortisol levels drop excessively, this will cause adrenal exhaustion.

So let's stop and look at the big picture.

If you have been diagnosed with hypothyroidism, then you'll recognize these symptoms: feeling cold and sluggish and having a slow metabolism. Now what comes next may surprise you, because most doctors won't discuss this. However, integrative physicians will tell you that if you have this diagnosis and are under physical and or emotional stress (and who isn't), then you are likely already in adrenal fatigue.

Here's why: Unrelenting stress during the early phases of adrenal fatigue generates excessive cortisol in the body, and this will negatively affect thyroid hormone production. How? Cortisol does this by suppressing the hypothalamus and the pituitary gland, which both control the thyroid. Therefore, it can induce an underactive thyroid—hypothyroidism.

So far, you can see how your thyroid, hormones, and adrenal glands are delicately intertwined like a spider web. It's difficult to see where one ends and the other starts, so in my opinion, it's insane to just treat a thyroid issue when there are so many other pieces that interconnect. Yet, most traditional doctors address only a few of these issues and then treat them separately.

There's one big piece to this puzzle we haven't even addressed: Mitochondria.

Your metabolism is your body's ability to create energy out of food. This is accomplished only through the mitochondria in your cells. The key to a healthy weight, therefore, is healthy mitochondria.

If you want to lose weight, you need your mitochondria to burn off fat.

Listen closely: The health of your mitochondria is dependent on the choices you make, including your food choices. Every time you spike your insulin (with processed food or sugars), you put your mitochondria health at risk.

Traditional medicine focuses on treatments and treating symptoms only. Having written thousands and thousands of weight-loss meal plans and coached just as many people for nearly a decade, it's my job to focus on the whole picture and manage the exceptions.

Together, you and I will work through the exceptions as we create your blueprint for success.

What I want you to remember is this: Everything is fixable. Your cells regenerate every day throughout the year. So now you have the opportunity for true wellness, weight loss, and healthy cells.

So let's begin to create your blueprint to success.

Chapter 12

Creating Your Blueprint to Success

You've heard the saying: A goal without a plan is only a wish!! Hang in there—the work you're doing now by reading this book and calculating your daily caloric and macronutrient goals means you will be wildly successful. I promise!

Earlier, we broke down the three essential macronutrients: lean protein, complex carbohydrates, and healthy fats. You can also find your foods broken out in the resource section of the book. Lean proteins, complex carbs, and healthy fats are the three macros you need to incorporate into your blueprint to success—not just calories. Calories will never tell the entire weight loss story, because all calories are NOT created equal.

As a rule (we'll talk about exceptions in upcoming chapters), you may want to consider a 40/40/20 breakdown of your macros:

40 percent of your diet should include lean protein

40 percent complex carbohydrates

20 percent healthy fats

This is the general rule that we follow for our #beMarthaFit clients and is a weight loss industry standard, so this may be your starting point as well.

Each macronutrient carries its own caloric level.

For example: Lean protein has 4 calories per gram, as do carbohydrates. Fat has 9 calories per gram.

Throughout your entire journey, you will always want to prioritize macros over calories. Many find this complicated, but prioritizing nutrients (which are macros) can help you make healthier food choices while fueling your body for the day. Always remember, not all calories are created equal, which is the biggest reason why we focus on macronutrients!

No matter which percentage you choose for your macronutrient levels, you will always want to prioritize lean protein. This macro should be the one you focus on prior to carbs or fats. Remember, protein is essential for your body to repair daily.

Now, you must prioritize an energy source. You have two energy source options: complex carbohydrates and healthy fats. Your body absolutely needs both, but choose one to be the dominant source, never both (carbohydrates and fats) at the same time. Choosing both at a high percentage level would mean that you'd have an energy excess, which would lead to weight gain.

The 40/40/20 split I have mentioned is a great place to begin, but as a long-time wellness and weight loss coach, I see many exceptions to this rule. As you can imagine, there is no one-size-fits-all approach to the inner workings of our body; therefore, I never take this approach to weight loss.

Coach Tip: Always remember to prioritize lean protein first. Then choose your energy source: complex carbohydrates or healthy fats. NEVER both.

Chapter 13

Creating Your Plan: Calculating Calories

Math is hard. I'm the running joke in the Kerr family. My father was a certified public accountant (CPA); my mother should have been a CPA; and my oldest sister, Deb, is a CPA. They are all math wizards. Me? Not so much. So I'm going to make the next two chapters as simple as possible, with as little math as possible. Because math is hard.

We will be calculating your daily calories in this chapter and then breaking down macros in the following chapter.

Deep breath. Let's get started!

There are dozens of caloric and macro calculators you will find on the internet. But just like everything else, you need to know how to cut through the misinformation and clutter.

The industry standard for calculations is the Harris-Benedict equation. This online calculator will do all the work for you. If you choose to use the Harris-Benedict equation, you'll notice it will deliver your BMR (basal metabolic rate) and TDE (total daily expenditure).

Here's your takeaway:

> Your BMR is the fuel you'd need daily if you slept all day long, did nothing, and were literally like a vegetable.
>
> Your TDE is what you burn through in a day and the number of calories you need to maintain your weight.

Keep in mind that the Harris-Benedict is an online calculator that doesn't take into consideration all the exceptions I mentioned in chapter 12—thyroid health, adrenal gland health, hormones, and mitochondria health. So proceed with caution.

It is widely known that if you reduce your daily caloric intake by approximately 500 calories a day, therefore eat 3,500 FEWER calories a week, you will lose between 1 to 2 pounds a week. This is a very safe weekly weight loss goal.

So, let's run an example client through the Harris-Benedict equation:

> Female, age 48
>
> Height: 6 feet
>
> Weight: 188 pounds
>
> Daily activity: Sedentary job, works out 3–4 times a week

According to the Harris-Benedict equation, her BMR is calculated at 1,597 (calories she needs to survive).

Her TDE is calculated to be 2,196 (calories, on average, that she burns daily).

After subtracting 500 calories a day (from her TDE number) for an entire week, this client's total daily calories for weight loss would be approximately 1,690. We never subtract from the BMR, as that is the fuel number your body needs just to sustain life.

Remember, the Harris-Benedict equation is simply a starting point to understand how many calories your body needs to live, to maintain, and to lose weight.

Many certified wellness and weight-loss coaches will tell you simply this:

Take your current weight.

Multiply it by 10.

Subtract 10–15 percent.

That number will be your caloric level for weight loss.

Let's run this simple equation for our example client above.

The female client weighs 188 pounds. Multiply by 10, and you have 1,880 calories. Now subtract 10 to 15 percent, and you have 1,692 to 1,598 calories for weight loss.

Why 10 to 15 percent? For my clients, I try to be as aggressive as possible, yet still retain optimum health, with their weekly weight loss. So, if possible, I try to reduce their daily calories by 15 percent. In most cases, that would net an average two-pound loss per week. However, based on client's health, daily activities, and workout schedule, there are times when I can reduce their calories by only 10 percent.

Now it's time for you to run your own numbers. I would suggest running the Harris-Benedict equation, and then you can run the simple equation I have provided. Compare the two sets of numbers.

Step 1: Take your current weight (ex: 200 pounds)

Step 2: Multiply your current weight by 10 (ex: 200 x 10 = 2,000 calories to maintain your current weight)

Step 3: Subtract 15 percent from your #2 answer (ex: 2,000 – 15 percent = 1,700)

As your wellness and weight loss coach, the first plan I would personally write for you would incorporate 1,700 calories. Now, the next step is vitally important: What will be the composition of the 1,700 calories you eat daily? As I continue to mention, not all calories are created equal.

In the next chapter, we will determine your macronutrient breakdown and start exploring foods.

Coach Tip: Always start by running your detailed information through the Harris-Benedict equation. Do not overestimate your daily activity on the calculator.

Chapter 14

Creating Your Plan: The Macro Breakdown

Throughout your weight loss journey, you will likely need to reference this and the previous chapter many times. Assuming you are consistently on-plan and losing weight, I recommend that you re-run your calories approximately every three to four weeks. This will ensure that you don't experience weight loss plateaus.

Let's continue to use our example client:

Female, age 48

Height: 6 feet

Weight: 188 pounds

Daily activity: Sedentary job, works out 3–4 times a week

Her BMR is calculated at 1,597

Her TDEE is calculated to be 2,196

Daily calories needed for weight loss: 1,690

Your next step is to divide the 1,690 calories by your preferred macronutrient split.

Remember we outlined the conventional 40/40/20 split as a fantastic starting point.

If we did our calculations, here is how our macronutrient split would look:

Calories: 1,690 daily
Protein (40 percent): 676 calories daily
Complex Carbs (40 percent): 676 calories daily
Fats (20 percent): 338 calories daily

Most clients succeed with eating five meals a day. This plan has you eating approximately every two to three hours, which will keep your blood sugar steady, and you will not "crash" or overeat from being overly hungry.

If you choose to eat five meals a day, you can, in this example, simply divide 1,690 by 5. This means for each meal, you would need to eat approximately 338 calories and would hit the following macros: protein (40 percent), 135 calories; complex carbs (40 percent), 135 calories; and fats (20 percent), 68 calories.

If you would rather divide this out by grams, you may. Remember, I told you that protein and complex carbs are 4 calories each. That means if we are aiming for 135 calories of protein and complex carbs, we need approximately 33 grams of each per meal. For fats, you will want to aim for approximately 8 grams per meal.

The easiest way to track your macronutrients throughout the day is to begin logging your foods in My Fitness Pal. As you log, you can check on your calories and macros to ensure you are hitting your 40/40/20 split. Additionally, by logging throughout your day, if you don't hit your caloric and macronutrient goal for one meal, you can "make it up" in the next.

For example: if your breakfast is lower than 338 calories, you would want to be deliberate about making up those calories in your morning snack or lunch.

The same applies to your macronutrient goals for each meal. If, for example, you don't hit your goal of 40/40/20 for your breakfast (perhaps you were short in protein), then aim to make that up in your next meal.

Always remember, protein is your priority, followed by one of your energy sources: complex carbs or fats. Not both.

You don't have to hit the 40/40/20 split for each meal, but focus on the entire day. Don't micro-manage every meal. Also realize that it's the net effect over a week. If you are consistently hitting (or are close to) your 40/40/20 split throughout the week, you will lose weight.

Coach Tip: Remember to focus on the whole day and not be obsessive about meeting your macro breakdown for each meal. It's the whole day that matters and the net effect over an entire week.

Chapter 15

Creating Your Plan: Reading Nutrition Labels

If it doesn't challenge you, it doesn't change you. I know these chapters are challenging. Keep pressing forward—you are so close to having your blueprint to success!

Pop-Tarts and oatmeal may have similar caloric levels, but the macronutrient breakdown for each is wildly different. As you move forward into creating your food plan and executing it long term, learning to read nutrition labels will become imperative. There's no way around it. So let's deep dive together.

By now you know the important macronutrients you need daily are protein, carbohydrates (complex), and fats. Each one of these macros is listed on every nutrition label. Additionally, you'll find micronutrients listed as well. For now, let's focus only on the macros.

Let's review this together.

> 1 Pop-Tart has 190 calories
> Protein: 2g
> Carbs: 37g
> Fats: 4g

Now let's remember our example client. She needs 1,690 calories daily to lose weight. This means she needs approximately 338 calories per meal with a 40/40/20 split. So she needs 33 grams of protein, 33 grams of complex carbs, and 9 grams of fat per meal.

You'll notice the carbs listed for ONE Pop-Tart are 37 grams. On the surface, this may seem acceptable. But notice what's missing? Protein. And remember, protein is always your first priority. Beyond repairing your body daily, protein will slow down the absorption of carbohydrates.

Sadly, there won't be any room in your food plan for something like a Pop-Tart. Beyond the fact that it doesn't support your macro split (lack of protein), the carbs in Pop-Tarts are simple, fast carbs—sugar. There is nothing complex about the ingredients in Pop-Tarts.

Now, let's look at a #beMarthaFit-approved recipe. Hopefully, this will satisfy any Pop-Tart craving you have.

Cinnamon Roll Coffee Cake

Nutrition facts (per serving):

> Calories: 106
> Protein: 12 g
> Carbs: 9 g
> Fat: 2 g

Look at this incredible recipe we have remastered in the #beMarthaFit Kitchen.

For your breakfast, you could eat three of these. A serving size of three would calculate to be: 318 calories, 36 grams of protein (perfection), 27 grams of carbs (again, very close to perfection), and 6 grams of fat.

Additionally, here are the ingredients. The full recipe is in the appendix:

 2 scoops vanilla protein powder
 1 cup Kodiak buttermilk pancake mix
 ⅔ cup nonfat yogurt
 2 large eggs
 ¼ cup sweetener (optional)
 1 tsp vanilla
 1 tbs sugar-free maple syrup

FILLING: 2 tbs swerve brown sugar and 1.5 tbs cinnamon

ICING: 1 tbs vanilla protein powder, 1 tbs whipped cream cheese, 1.5 tbs cashew milk, 1 tbs swerve confectionery sugar

You have a protein-packed, complex carbohydrate, low-fat breakfast recipe that will absolutely meet your caloric and macronutrient goals.

So as you begin to populate your meal plan with whole foods, single-ingredient foods, foods from a mother, you will need to be highly aware of nutrition labels.

Coach Tip: Stop concentrating solely on the number of calories a food has. Look deeper into what composes those calories. Focus on protein first, followed by an energy source—carbs or fats. Never both.

Chapter 16

Creating Your Plan: Choosing Your Foods

You are embarking on a journey that literally has you unlearning what you thought you knew. Learn to unlearn, and through that, learn to be comfortable outside of your comfort zone. I'm always here as your guide, but remember, the execution is solely reliant on you.

Whole foods.

Nutrient-dense foods.

Single-ingredient foods.

Foods from a mother.

If you've never explored the world of "clean eating" or "macro-based meal plans," these terms may sound foreign to you, so let me help you define each.

Whole Foods. These are foods that have been refined or processed very little. They are generally free of additives and preservatives and include beans, fruits, vegetables, seeds, and nuts.

Nutrient-Dense Foods. Nutrient dense simply means you are giving your body the fuel that it needs without a ton of extra calories. You can add lean protein to this list and include all the foods we mentioned under Whole Foods.

Single-Ingredient Foods. I want you to focus on finding foods that literally have one ingredient in them. Very few, if any, packaged foods will have a single ingredient in them. For example, examine a bag of prepared chicken breasts at the grocery store. If you look beyond the nutrition label and farther down into the list of ingredients, you will likely find much more listed than JUST the chicken breasts. Why? Because it's been bagged in the freezer section, you will find it contains additives and preservatives. The better choice is simply to grab the chicken from the butcher.

Foods from a Mother. Here's a simple visual: eggs come from a chicken— food from a mother. Vegetables can easily fall from this category as well— foods from the "mother" vine.

These definitions all have a similar thread. Nothing is overly processed or full of artificial flavors or additives; foods are fresh(er); they are not pre-packaged; they have very few ingredients (so your body can process what you have eaten); and to be very blunt, the food is real!

Eat real food!

This means the days of grab and go, drive-thrus, and microwaved pre-packaged meals are done, for the most part. Often, you will avoid these traps and truly focus on whole foods, nutrient-dense foods, single-ingredient foods, and foods from a mother.

You may be wildly overwhelmed. I get it. Most clients of #beMarthaFit are overwhelmed when they begin. You're learning something new and undoing the shopping habits you have had for years!! Take your time learning the #beMarthaFit way, and remember that no one expects you to be perfect right out of the gate, nor will your journey be perfect.

Now that you know your caloric and macronutrient breakdown, you have an entire day to fill with yummy foods. I want to give you a jumpstart and provide you with a sample Healthy Eating Blueprint, which you will find in the appendix of this book. Remember, it's important that you log your foods into My Fitness Pal so that you are reaching your daily caloric and macronutrient goals. Adjust your portions accordingly. Also in the appendix are a few examples of meal plans with a 40/40/20 split that we have outlined.

Remember, eating this way should NOT be boring or limiting. I have shared several recipes in the appendix to get you started. Additionally, we have hundreds and hundreds of recipes on our subscription recipe website. Details for this are also in the appendix. Here you can access recipes for all meals and snacks. Each recipe includes calories and macros for ease of use. As you think about the foods you want to eat and explore recipes, rest assured that you will find so many of your favorites, but they have been "remastered" to be macronutrient balanced and low calorie. Keep an open mind as you hunt down new ingredients and take a new mindset approach toward what you're eating.

Lastly, remember to reference the "Yes, No, Maybe" list of foods in the appendix.

Coach Tip: When you get time, assess the sauces and spices you are using. Your spices may be LOADED with sodium. Start exploring lower-sodium options. In general, you will want to keep your sodium at about 2,500 mg a day. Ditch the table salt and instead use pink Himalayan salt. Your table salt has been bleached and offers no micronutrient value. Pink sea salt, on the other hand, is full of the micronutrients you need. If you are a woman with a thyroid issue, you absolutely should be using pink salt, as an iodine deficiency also occurs with hypothyroidism. The natural iodine in pink salt assists your body in synthesizing thyroid hormones.

When it comes to sauces, you'll notice most of them are full of sugar. This isn't necessary for flavor and will very quickly add up in wasted calories. In the appendix, I have included an exhaustive list of #beMarthaFit-approved sauces. You will be amazed at the flavors without the added sugar and calories.

Chapter 17

Creating Your Plan: Adjusting Macros for Hormone Issues and Health Diagnosis

Everyone's body is wildly different, just like snowflakes. No two are ever alike. While you may look like your siblings or have a similar height and body structure as a close friend, you are wildly different on the inside. For this very reason, there cannot be a one-size-fits-all approach to weight loss, and managing exceptions is vital.

We've outlined the widely used 40/40/20 split of protein, complex carbs, and healthy fats. This is one approach to ensuring your macronutrient needs, but it's important to know that not every woman will respond well to this split. Therefore, you may be frustrated with the lack of weight loss!

After writing customized meal plans for nearly a decade and seeing how hormones can wreak havoc on the weight loss process, it's vitally important to discuss this very issue.

Starting in the mid-forties, most women's bodies become a war of hormones. Whether you're close to menopause or not, your hormones begin to fluctuate very irregularly. What generally occurs is women have too much estrogen and too little progesterone. You may feel "off" or you may feel perfectly normal, as I did. Simply said, this is the time when egg production dwindles, and hormones take on a life of their own.

Additionally, during this time, many women become increasingly insulin resistant. But insulin resistance doesn't just strike women in their forties and above. Insulin resistance comes with many other conditions such as PCOS (polycystic ovarian syndrome) and obesity, and habits such as lack of exercise, smoking, and even lack of sleep. And like I said, you don't have to be in your forties to be insulin resistant. I see many teens and young women in their twenties dealing with this. Also note, you do NOT have to be diabetic to be dealing with insulin resistance.

So, what does this mean for weight loss?

Everything!

Estrogen dominance, and therefore not enough progesterone, leads to a whole host of chronic illnesses, and it means you have an insulin resistance issue, which is likely part of your weight issue.

When you are insulin resistant, it means your cells don't respond properly to the hormone insulin.

If your doctor told you that you are insulin resistant, then your doctor would also tell you to avoid overly processed foods, sugary foods, and carbohydrates. Reducing carb intake reduces the amount of insulin circulating in the body, and this works to reduce insulin resistance.

But for the sake of your journey, let's take this one step further. Rather than implementing the traditional 40/40/20 split of protein, complex carbs, and healthy fats, we are going to reverse your energy source.

Your 40/40/20 macronutrient split will be changed to 40 percent protein, 40 percent HEALTHY FATS, and 20 percent complex carbs.

Complex carbs are not the enemy, but your body, due to your hormones, will be better served with fewer carbohydrates and more healthy fats. Your primary energy source will be fats, followed up with a small amount of complex carbs. Remember, your protein level is still appropriately high.

Whether you know that you are estrogen dominant or if you have been diagnosed as insulin resistant, there is no harm in executing the above-mentioned macro breakdown and having healthy fats as your primary energy source. Just note that you may not have an instant feeling of being full, as you would with complex carbs. Additionally, watch your portion sizes with your healthy fats. There is a tendency to over-eat healthy fats—they taste so good!

Coach Tip: If you are a woman in your mid-forties or older, or you have been diagnosed as insulin resistant or with PCOS, start with this macro breakdown:

40 percent lean protein

40 percent healthy fats

20 percent complex carbs

Chapter 18

Exploring Carb Cycling

My job is to be your guide and have you focus on one thing at a time. So remember this we explore carb cycling and intermittent fasting (next chapter). The quickest way to get overwhelmed is to add too many things too fast. I want you to be slow and deliberate with your journey. Do one thing at a time.

Carb cycling is an eating plan that cycles through low-carb and higher-carb days. Most athletes will carb cycle and include higher-carb days when they plan tougher workouts. But you don't have to be an athlete to implement carb cycling. You, for example, could plan a higher carb day on the days you work out and lower carb days on your rest days. Remember, the point of eating carbohydrates is for energy, and you need more energy on your workout days versus your off days or days when you're sitting most of the day.

If you choose to implement carb cycling as part of your meal plan, please know there are so many variations to execute, but your main goal is to properly drain excess glycogen (energy) storage on low carb days and fuel your workouts with high carb days, which in turn will fill up your energy "bucket."

The good news is you have options!

One day low carb, next day high carb, then repeat.

Two days low carb, one day high carb, then repeat.

Or schedule your high carb days on your intense workout days and remain low carb the other days.

There's no wrong way to execute carb cycling. The important factor to remember is when you are executing a low-carb day, your body is relying on stored fat for energy. Additionally, on low-carb days, your energy source will be healthy fats. On high-carb days, your energy source is complex carbs (therefore low fat), and you will be using the glycogen from the carbs for energy.

Keep in mind that when you execute carb cycling, you are also manipulating your insulin levels, and for this very reason, it can be a solid option for those who are diagnosed with insulin resistance. Low-carb days keep the insulin levels low. Higher-carb days rev up your metabolism.

Here's a good starting point:

> Eat an average of 80 grams of carbs for low-carb days. This means your fat grams will be much higher as healthy fats are your energy source this day.

> Eat an average of 150+ grams of carbs for higher-carb days. This means your fat grams will be very low, and carbs are now your energy source for the day.

NOTE: if you are insulin resistant, take note of how you feel on high-carb days. You may gradually, need to reduce your allotted grams of carbs, but do that slowly. Your body absolutely needs this energy source.

When you begin carb cycling, keep your carbs below 100 grams for low-carb days. If you are insulin resistant and choose carb cycling, take note of how you feel on your high-carb days.

Carb cycling is also ideal when you are on a weight-loss plateau. Remember you always want to be in a caloric deficit, but if you feel you have been "stuck" at the same weight for more than two weeks, temporarily implementing carb cycling can propel you to a new, lower weight.

There is no one way to execute carb cycling, which can make it tricky and perhaps frustrating for anyone to execute. There can be a lot of fine tuning to do, which can lead to confusion. I highly suggest you experiment with the high-carb days throughout the week. For many of our clients, we immediately start them out on a 2:1 protocol: two low-carb days followed by one higher-carb day and repeat. For most of our clients, this nets a favorable weight-loss result. However, occasionally, we up their low-carb days to three, followed by one high-carb day. You will need to experiment and be aware of how you feel throughout your low- and higher-carb days.

Remember, on high carb days, you must fuel yourself with complex carbs. Refer to the list of complex carbs in the appendix. This is not an all-out Pop-Tart fest.

Coach Tip: In the appendix, I have included an example carb cycling meal plan. Use this plan as a guide to create your own personal carb cycling plan.

Chapter 19

Introducing Intermittent Fasting

What if I told you intermittent fasting was really intermittent eating?? Would it sound easier and "less bad" that way? Sometimes we must flip the script we are telling ourselves. Intermittent fasting doesn't mean skipping meals; it simply means delaying your first meal and eating all your meals within an eating window!

Intermittent fasting is wildly popular, and rightfully so, as it provides a wealth of health benefits. Intermittent fasting is cycling through periods of eating and then fasting. The goal of intermittent fasting is to increase the health and function of your cells, genes, and hormones to access your fat cells easily and promote weight loss.

When you fast, your insulin levels drop and human growth hormone increases. These two functions will innately lead to the breakdown of your body's fat cells to use fat for energy, and this will net you a solid weight loss.

By fasting for long periods (often sixteen hours, which includes sleep), it allows our body's insulin/sugar levels to drop, and this allows our fat cells to be accessed, to release energy, and therefore to burn fat. And therefore, if you're insulin resistant or pre-diabetic, intermittent fasting is beneficial.

In nearly a decade of coaching, we have found the easiest and most highly effective way to execute intermittent fasting is with the 16:8 protocol. This means you will eat all your meals within eight hours and fast for sixteen, which, as I have stated, includes your sleep. During your sixteen hours of fasting, you may drink water, black coffee, and tea. We advise our clients to use very little to no half-and-half, sugar-free creamer, and artificial sweetener during fasting hours.

As you proceed through your sixteen-hour fast, your body is doing some amazing work, all for you.

Between hours four and six, your blood sugar levels are reducing; food has left the stomach and insulin is no longer being produced.

Close to the twelve-hour mark of fasting, your food has been burned for energy, your digestive system begins to rest, your body heals, and human growth hormone (HGH) increases.

In hours fourteen to sixteen, your body has begun to use fat as energy, your HGH rapidly increases, and your body is ramping up fat burning.

During hours eighteen to twenty-four, human growth hormone starts to soar, autophagia begins, your glycogen is drained, and ketones are released into the bloodstream.

I keep mentioning human growth hormone (HGH). This is produced by the pituitary glands and spurs growth in children and teens. But it also helps regulate body composition, body fluids, muscle and bone growth, sugar, and fat metabolism. You will find tons of articles on boosting your HGH naturally. The very first way to boost your HGH will be to lose body fat, and the second way is to fast intermittently. I tell you this, so you can trust the process and journey you have embarked upon.

After fasting for sixteen hours and enjoying water, coffee, or tea, you will break your fast and eat accordingly to your plan. This is not a time for a treat meal. Eat only the foods on your plan.

The 16:8 intermittent fasting protocol is an easy one to manage. It literally fits into anyone's schedule. Do not get legalistic with this. If by chance one day you only fast for fifteen hours, you're fine. If by chance you need to shift your eating hours, you will also be fine. Nothing about intermittent fasting should feel rigid. Remember, it's the net effect over a week. And to be super transparent, if you have one day where you do not implement 16:8, you will also be fine.

Periodically, in our #beMarthaFit programs, I will have clients execute a twenty-four-hour fast. A twenty-four-hour fast should be done with purpose and intent, not just because you feel like it. Here are a few reasons to execute this extended fast:

1. Weight loss plateaus and you are not at all hungry. A twenty-four-hour fast, of course, will put you in a deeper caloric deficit.

2. Fasting for longer periods can allow your body to repair and "fix" the effects of everyday damage.

3. Some will say that it renews your immune system. This happens because stem cells start producing white blood cells when you stop eating.

Proceed with caution with a twenty-four-hour fast. Have a specific reason for doing it.

Our goal is for you enjoy eating, to not be afraid of eating, and to eat to fuel your body. I get concerned when someone is doing an extended fast just because they think it will help them. Remember, food is fuel, and a twenty-four-hour fast should be done with care and purpose.

When you end your twenty-four-hour fast, you eat according to plan. As with most of my clients, that means you will eat one or two meals. Most clients break their fast with their dinner; some break it slightly earlier and have their afternoon snack and a later dinner. Then they immediately begin again with the 16:8 protocol.

After a twenty-four-hour fast, for some clients, it's a great time to incorporate a treat meal. If you do this, choose wisely. Often when a client has a treat meal, it ends up being a treat day or even worse, a treat weekend. I have no issues with a treat meal after a twenty-four-hour fast, but how you handle yourself after the treat meal is of utmost importance.

If you choose a treat meal to break your twenty-four-hour fast, allow yourself approximately 1,000 calories for this meal if you're a woman and about 1,800 calories if you're a man. You won't necessarily need to count your macros for this treat meal; however, you must still prioritize lean protein, followed by ONE energy source: complex carbs or fats. NOT BOTH.

Only you can determine if you feel strong enough to go off-plan and have a treat meal without guilt, without shame, and with the ability to get back on plan immediately. So really think this through and plan accordingly.

We will break out the role of treat meals in Section 3 of the book.

Coach Tip: Implement your 16:8 protocol for as long as possible and reserve your twenty-four-hour fasts when you hit a weight loss plateau.

Chapter 20

The Water Game

Every single day, I line up my water bottles. For me, it's a game, and I hope you will take the same fun approach. My mother, who is in her mid-eighties, thinks she has this game mastered. She tells me she drinks several glasses of water a day. We have had this conversation multiple times. It goes like this: "Mom, you aren't drinking enough water, and it's going to start affecting every area of your life."

Last year, she was having dizzy spells every day, she was feeling weak and rundown, and honestly, it got to a point where we were all highly concerned, and she saw her doctor. Do you want to know the reason she felt like this? She was severely dehydrated. Very honestly, I laughed. I wasn't shocked, but she needed to hear this from her doctor, not her daughter who specializes in this. Every time I tell this story, I have a good laugh.

Let's start by discussing why your body needs water, and then we'll break out how much.

Every part of your body uses water—-organs, cells, and tissue. Your body uses water to regulate its temperature and maintain bodily functions. Your body is continually losing water to digestion, sweating, and even breathing. Your body is composed of 60 percent water, the brain and heart are approximately 73 percent water, and your lungs are about 83 percent water. No wonder my mother Lynn was feeling horrible! Her three or four 8-ounce glasses of water a day weren't cutting it.

I'm hopeful you can see why your body needs to be continually hydrated. It craves water, not juices or sodas. Pure water.

But does water really assist in weight loss?

One hundred percent yes!

The short answer is, drinking water will boost your metabolism, aid in digestion, cleanse your body of waste, and act as an appetite suppressant. Also remember that water flushes water. So drinking more water will help your body stop water retention, which has historically led to inflammation in your body.

The great debate lies with how much water you need.

As a master wellness and weight loss coach, I tell my clients to drink a gallon of water a day. Now, I know that sounds like a lot, and it is, but I will also tell you that when clients consistently fall short in their water intake, it affects their weigh-ins every single week. As soon as they up their water game back to 128 ounces a day, they lose weight.

Trusted sources such as WebMD will outline that you should be drinking between a half ounce and a full ounce of water per pound that you weigh. For example, according to WebMD, someone who weighs 150 pounds should be drinking approximately 75 to 150 ounces a day.

That is a wide range: 75 to 150 ounces a day!

As I have mentioned before, I like to be as healthfully aggressive as possible with our weight loss clients. So, keeping that in mind, I push our clients to drink one gallon a day, and when they do, they see an increase in their weight loss, week by week.

Drinking water throughout the day is not a race. It's vitally important that you don't rush to finish your gallon by early morning or even lunch time. Flushing too much water into your body too quickly will lead to an electrolyte and sodium imbalance, which can lead to water intoxication. This is a very real and very serious issue, but it should not scare anyone from being properly hydrated.

A safe way to attack your daily water intake is to drink half a gallon by lunch time and the other half in the afternoon.

Coach Tip: Drink the water and know that your body is thanking you. And if you want to join me with my daily water game, get yourself the seventeen-ounce water bottles from the grocery store. Line up eight of them every day. Plan to finish four by lunch time and then other four in the afternoon.

Chapter 21

The New Car Syndrome

Every single client I work with is ready to start yesterday. They are on fire, and they are eager and ready to start their customized plan immediately. They dig in, get to the grocery store, ask a million questions, participate in our VIP Client Group Page for support, and see amazing results.

And then, the fire fades.

We'll call this the new car syndrome. You purchase a new or pre-owned car, you wash it every day, you freak if someone spills something, you garage the car, and you vacuum it weekly.

Then, the newness wears off, and now you have trash, empty water bottles, dirt, sand, and dog hair in what used to be your newly prized possession. Hey, I'm guilty as well.

The newness has worn off. Now it's just another chore.

Ah, friend, I hate to break it to you, but this is exactly how you will feel at some point about your meal plan and your journey!

One of the very reasons we provide updated food plans to our full-time clients is to avoid boredom (and make sure they don't hit a long-term weight loss plateau). I find around the three- to four-week mark, clients need a shake-up, new options, new meals, something fresh. You will, too.

But let's go further out in your journey. As a coach to thousands, I see a trend. After the twelve-week mark, about 50 percent of our client's efforts start to decline. The newness of this way of eating has worn off. They've lost weight, some have gotten a little too confident, and soon the weight loss stales. It nets frustration, and sometimes they quit. My heart breaks when this happens. I know they will return later as a client, at a higher weight than when they left.

Hey, nothing is new forever. If you're in a relationship or marriage, you know this. The infatuation wanes, and you are left to do work to not only maintain the relationship, but also to grow it. Welcome to life. Why would your meal plan be any different? It's unrealistic to expect it to be fun and exciting every single month. But ask yourself this: when your marriage becomes boring, do you walk out? I would hope not. So then, why would you abandon your blueprint to success, which ultimately provides you with incredible health?

It's going to happen. You will be bored or overly confident in the weight loss you have realized. The new car syndrome is inevitable. You've been warned, sweet friend.

So how do you address or even fix this?

Most importantly, you must know and accept that it's going to happen. When it happens, ask yourself WHY you are bored? What would make this more fun? Often this issue is quickly fixed by changing up morning and afternoon snack options or even your breakfast choices. If this doesn't cause you to engage more with your incredible plan, perhaps you need a planned treat meal. We discuss this in a later chapter.

I hate the over-used saying: "Find your why!" However, the premise behind it is solid. We weren't created to just survive this life we were living; we were put on Earth to thrive. So referencing the concept of finding your "why" often allows us to remember WHY we started this wellness journey. But simply telling clients to "find their why" when the new car syndrome has occurred, or even worse, if they are apathetic about it all, doesn't work for many. Everyone needs action steps.

As a coach, I want to get my clients "unstuck"! What I mean is, once the new car syndrome strikes, clients are stuck in an internal battle of tension, knowing they really don't want to do the work, yet they have no real idea of what they want to do next. They are stuck between two choices, and frankly, two lives. It's a choice between living a life that leads to confidence, self-love, and assuredness or one that is like everyone else around them, eating and drinking according to their own whims. It's like clients are stuck in purgatory.

You know deep down that you are meant for more, but you are either scared of the work ahead of you, or frankly, you just don't want to do the work. Yikes!! Are you doomed? No! Not at all.

Let's attack this together:

Step 1: Admit it. Admit you are bored, tired, frustrated, or lacking motivation. You are restless. Do some soul searching as to exactly how you feel. If you prefer to really break this out and get your thoughts out of your head (which I advise), write it down. It's good to have this written down so you can perhaps find a trend as you proceed in your journey.

Step 2: Write exactly what you want right now. Maybe you want bread. Maybe you want a glass of wine, or the whole bottle. Maybe you want sleep. Or maybe you'd like a bowl of real, creamy ice cream. Maybe you need a day or two off-plan. Yes, I said that, because at times it's the truth. Now write down how you would feel if you indulged in any of the above. Get detailed with this step. How do you think you would feel? Would you be able to get back on plan? Would a few days off-plan mean you would struggle to engage again? Get detailed here. One-word answers aren't acceptable.

Step 3: Now say these words out loud: "I am not stuck!" That's right, you really aren't stuck; you simply need further direction. You need permission to have a treat meal, and frankly, you need something to look forward to. Remember, nothing stays new forever.

I can honestly tell you I still periodically have the new car syndrome. I hate it. But I recognize it just as I see how my marriage waxes and wanes. It's life. When I execute Step 3, I do this by looking at myself in the mirror. I really take time to look at me and repeatedly say out loud, "I am not stuck!" Note that this supports our positive self-talk, visualization, and manifestation. Imagine if I spent time looking in the mirror and saying, "You're stuck!" You clearly know what would happen next: self-sabotage.

A word of warning: If you started your journey for someone else, as soon as new car syndrome occurs, this is where you will quit. You will struggle with self-doubt, and you no longer will feel compelled to do the work, even if it means a small sacrifice.

Step 4: Now reflect and answer these questions:

Does your food plan provide stability for you during the daily chaos of life?

Have you experienced a higher level of confidence while on plan?

Do you have less anxiety and/or depression when you're on plan?

How do you feel about yourself when you look in the mirror, now that you are smaller and leaner?

How do you physically feel? How do your joints feel? Do you still have headaches?

How do you feel when you wake up in the morning? Are you refreshed and eager to start the day?

How do you feel when you see the results of your behaviors and choices and the scale goes down?

Step 4 requires self-reflection. A lot of how you are feeling is hidden in patterns of thoughts, behaviors, new habits, and feelings. You will not be able to proceed consistently with your meal plan if you haven't taken the time to self-reflect here.

If you find it hard to execute these four steps, then I highly advise you talk to a licensed therapist.

Remember, the best way to execute Steps 1 through 4 is by journaling. Now listen, I hate journaling. I'm not going lie to you. However, I will take fifteen minutes and work through Steps 1 through 4 on a piece of paper, because I always uncover what I need and how I feel, and I'm then able to better engage with my plan and set new goals. Yes, even in maintenance-mode, I still work through these steps (and you will, too), because every single time I do, I learn more about my choices and behaviors!

Ok, Steps 1 through 4 are done. You have defined how you feel and what you want, you've looked in the mirror and said out loud, "I am not stuck," and you've analyzed how you feel when you are following your meal plan. So now what? If you need a treat meal, refer to Chapter 23. If you feel you need a few days off-plan, do so, but with extreme caution. Make sure you will be able to "flip the switch" and get back on plan. No one can do that for you. Remember, no one is coming to save you or do this for you.

If you feel you need something to look forward to, start by changing the rotation of snacks and breakfast options you are offering yourself. Go back to our recipe website (listed in the appendix) or try a recipe in this book that you haven't before. Additionally, you may want to consider now implementing carb cycling or intermittent fasting. Trust me, there is always an answer, if you care to seek it out.

As a coach, you know I try to be on plan as much as possible; however, even in maintenance, I find that I need one event a month that I can look forward to. Sometimes it's an overnight girls' trip with a friend and I am off-plan. Or Stephen and I plan thirty days of being on plan and alcohol-free, and then we schedule an off-plan event together that will include foods we think we miss and a few adult beverages. This may be something you need to do, too. I will caution you, though: I feel comfortable executing events like this because I know I can immediately flip the switch and be back on plan. Even my clients have commented they have never seen someone get back on plan so fast. If you choose this method to refresh you, just make sure you are strong enough to be back on plan the very next meal or day. Yes, there are times throughout the year that you should not focus on your meal plan. Remember, this isn't a diet—this is a lifestyle. Not every day has to be the same, and you should focus on family and fellowship on holidays, birthdays, or other important events. But remember, you are responsible for "flipping the switch" and getting back to your lifestyle meal plan.

Remember, you always have options. You are never stuck. But don't avoid these four steps if the new car syndrome has smacked you in the face.

Chapter 22

Navigating the Grey

In 2016, during my twenty-two-week preparation for my first body-building competition, I was extremely legalistic. I had to be. You cannot get on stage deconditioned, and conditioning comes from food. There wasn't any wiggle room. There were hard deadlines (competition dates), so everything was black and white. Greys didn't exist. They couldn't exist, or I would not have gotten on stage.

Your long-term success in every area of your life will be learning to navigate the greys. If you only see black and white, good or bad, you will fall on your face and be continually disappointed in yourself or others. Grace simply doesn't exist in a black-and-white world.

The black-and-white mentality feeds into food categories: good and bad. Spoiler alert—you will never heal your relationship with food if you continue to look at food as good and bad.

Remember, I've told you there are times for off-plan meals and alcohol. At the beginning of your journey, that is not the time to navigate greys; that is the time to be legalistic. You are in a period of undoing the damage you have done, you are breaking free from old habits, you are allowing your body to trust you with your food choices, and in turn, your body will begin to work for you. If you were a full-time client, I would urge you to be as black and white as possible for the first twelve weeks. During the first twelve weeks, we aren't necessarily labeling some foods and alcohol as "bad." We are avoiding trigger foods and alcohol to maximize your results and banish cravings.

Then, we learn to navigate the grey.

Navigating the grey is recognizing that you need to learn to own the "space" between legalism and food freedom. Sweet friend, this is difficult and will take time, just like your journey. You will stumble a lot here, but that's awesome. Each time you stumble, you will learn more about yourself, your choices, and your behaviors.

Foods should never be put into "good" or "bad" buckets. When you categorize like this and choose a food from your "bad bucket," you will feel as if you did something bad. This is not a successful way to live life. As soon as you do this, you will feel immense guilt, shame, and anxiety over your decisions. If this happens to you, I want you to go to the mirror, look at yourself, and say this out loud: "I have done nothing wrong." Say that repeatedly throughout the day.

"I have done nothing wrong."

You haven't. You must show yourself grace right now and focus forward.

Navigating the greys is not intuitive. We were taught early on that our childhood decisions were either good or bad, and we were punished for the bad. So we continue this cycle into our adulthood. Teaching a child to navigate greys is extremely difficult when you are trying to instill that there are consequences for each action.

The first time I vividly remember navigating greys and learning grace was through my divorce. I had sought wise counsel from both a licensed family therapist and my church pastor and truly had their "permission" and understanding as to why I was leaving my first husband. But I had "friends" around me who thought otherwise.

These "friends" (and yes, it's purposeful that I have that word in quotations) were downright pushy, rude, and demeaning. They approached me with legalistic ideology, telling me I was ruining my first husband, and my young children would amount to nothing, all due to my separating and divorcing. One even threatened me, telling me that my oldest son had a higher calling, which would not be realized if I left my husband.

The reality of my first marriage and the depths to which it was broken meant that for me to survive, I had to leave. Either I would end up taking my own life, or I had to escape and rebuild.

In my church, my "friends" treated me as if I had a contagious disease, and if they remained friends with me, they too would catch it. So out came what I call "the Christian Lysol can," and I was unfriended, banished, and left alone. Still to this day, these "friends" have nothing to do with me. And you know what? That's okay. We are meant to lose the friends we were meant to lose. What I was doing was making them feel incredibly uncomfortable.

It was during this crisis time that I realized so much of how we operate is through black-and-white lenses, and that people truly have no grace for themselves, others, and others' choices that don't exactly line up with their own.

If you are believer, you know the ultimate grace-giver is Jesus. Even nailed to the cross, he was offering grace to those who wronged him. So it's astonishing to me that people feel the need to be so legalistic, to apply judgment, and to fail in listening to others.

The very same principle applies to your decision to put foods into the "good and bad" buckets.

This is extremely hard for a perfectionist to navigate; trust me, as a recovering perfectionist, I understand. So, if you categorize yourself as a perfectionist, then you likely feel you are either good or bad, right or wrong, perfect or completely off base and failing. Greys do not exist in your life.

Remember, none of this is intuitive, and I'm forcing you to learn to appreciate and navigate the grey areas of your food plan.

Immediately banish the theory that foods are either good or bad. There is a time for both. There is a time to make memories versus counting macronutrients. I would never tell a client not to partake, for example, at their adult child's wedding. To some extent, this can also be an approach to vacations.

Strike the balance. Once you get through your first twelve weeks of boot camp (aka your food plan), you should be actively working on striking the balance; for some, this will be a 90/10 or 80/20 approach.

The 90/10 or 80/20 approach simply means you will be on plan 80 or 90 percent of the time and allow for off-plan moments and events 10 to 20 percent of the time. Only you can determine your sweet-spot percentage. When I executed the 80/20 approach, I found my choices were turning into me executing the plan more like 60/40. That wasn't good enough for me while I wanted to lose, and it still wouldn't work for me in maintenance. I am comfortable navigating a 90/10 approach. You decide which approach to take, try it out, see how your behaviors and choices line up percentagewise, and adjust, like I did, if needed.

After your first twelve weeks, experiment first with the 90/10 approach. You can implement these two ways, and only you will know, based on your choices and behaviors, which is best. The first way to execute this is to allow yourself 10 percent off-plan each week. This likely means a reasonable weekly treat meal. In total transparency, this doesn't work for me. I get out with my husband, and I want to stay out, have more fun, drink more, and eat more pizza. You get the point.

So here is the second option: after many times of experimenting, I find it's best for me and many of my clients to enjoy the 10 percent off-plan just once a month. This way, if I need to shed a few pounds, or if my clients want to still realize a weight loss each week, they can, because they are allowing 10 percent off-plan only one time each month. During the 10 percent off-plan time, approach it with moderation.

As your guide, I highly suggest you begin to execute the 90/10 principle once a month to start. Note how you feel and how it affects your weight loss, and be mindful of your choices when off-plan. However, if you find yourself spending time self-loathing and downright beating yourself up, remind yourself of this: You have done nothing wrong!

Chapter 23

The Role of Treat Meals

Be careful how you word certain things. Certain words falsely and subconsciously lead us to believing we are failing! Any time a client references a cheat meal, I quickly correct them.

I am positive you have heard the term "cheat meal."

I hate it.

I hate the word "cheat"!

By now, you know that this journey is equal parts food and your mentality. So if we use the word "cheat," that signals something bad—bad behavior, bad choice. Let's set the record straight: this is not going to be a cheat meal, but rather a treat meal.

Treat meals absolutely serve a purpose. As I've mentioned before, I think you should avoid a treat meal within your first twelve weeks of your journey. Remember you are paving a road to a new life, and your mindset and willpower aren't strong enough to indulge within the first twelve weeks.

Treat meals are fabulous for many reasons:

Too much deprivation can then lead to bingeing

Treat meals, if done correctly, can boost your metabolism in the short term

They allow you to enjoy foods that you have cut from your life, in moderation

They allow for participation in some social events that you may have avoided

You're likely wondering how to execute your treat meal without it turning into a cheat day, week, or even worse, month. Yes, I've had clients who can't find their footing for a month when they loosen the reigns.

Step 1: Allow yourself to accept that a treat meal will not ruin your long-term progress. One off-plan meal will not negate all the good you have done. You should not have anxiety or fear for going off-plan. Remember, this is part of learning how to navigate the grey. You are doing nothing wrong by having a treat meal.

Step 2: Plan! Do not be spontaneous with your treat meal. Plan it, look forward to it, and most importantly, before you leave your house, decide exactly what you are craving. Do not step outside your front door until you have a plan in place. What will you eat? How long will you stay? Is alcohol involved? If you don't plan it out before leaving, your treat meal will lead to a treat experience; you'll end up staying out longer, perhaps bar-hopping, and soon you will have had a food festivus. This isn't a treat meal.

Step 3: Pick your poison! I write that with a smile on my face; you can't have it all. This isn't a gorge fest. Most importantly, you need to pick which you want more: off-plan foods or alcohol. Don't try and navigate both. Every-thing gets muddy when you combine off-plan foods and alcohol. Frankly, once you pass the two-drink limit, you'll likely be making poor choices, including what you continue to eat.

If you choose both a high-carbohydrate off-plan meal and sugary alcoholic drinks, you will "spill over." What does this mean? "Spilling over" means you will have ingested too many carbohydrates and sugar, your glycogen storage (think of it as a bucket filling up) will be in excess (the bucket spills over), and you will be bloated, having a large amount of subcutaneous water (under your skin). It will take several days for your body to push out the excess, and you will likely feel miserable—your joints will ache and you'll likely have a blasted headache.

This is exactly why I say, pick your poison. Pick one—off-plan foods or alcohol, but not both.

What's important to remember is how you handle yourself after your planned treat meal. This is where the rubber meets the road. Immediately you must get back on your plan and immediately return to drinking your gallon of water, daily.

What NOT to do: Do not feel guilty. You have done nothing wrong. Remind yourself of this! You had one treat meal, and this is an important phase of your journey that you must learn to navigate. Do not starve yourself or punish yourself for eating off-plan. This is counterintuitive to your learning process. Additionally, do not go do a long workout to "make up" for having the off-plan foods.

All you must do is get back on plan immediately. Eat all the food on your plan and drink your water. It's really that simple.

So what should you do if your planned treat meal turned into a treat day, weekend, or longer? Don't worry; we'll discuss that soon.

Chapter 24

The Role of Alcohol

I get the funniest emails at times. About once a week, someone inquires about a consult call, and in the email, the client asks if he or she can drink on the weekends and still lose weight. I giggle every time. I always feel this prospective client is asking me for permission. Am I going to say yes? No. Flat-out no. I'm not going to give a client permission to drink alcohol consistently. But before you throw this book at the wall and scream my name, let me drop a few truth bombs on you.

Am I saying you can never drink alcohol again? No.

Now is not the time, however.

Right now, you are trying to break old habits, years of old habits. By reaching for a bottle of wine or a beer, you are continually taking steps back to your old life. Your habits of reaching for alcohol at the end of the day, or on Friday afternoons and into the weekends, are learned behavior choices.

Remember Pavlov's dogs? The premise behind his experiment was that objects or events could trigger a conditioned response in his dogs. Pavlov's experiments started by demonstrating how the presence of a bowl of dog food (stimulus) would trigger a conditioned response of salivation.

Yes, we should consider our human tastes more discerning that those of a pet, but research from Scientific American shows that humans can be trained to crave food (or alcohol in this example) in a manner reminiscent of Pavlov's dogs.

I know this will sound super basic, but follow me here: walking in the door from work and opening a beer or pouring yourself a glass of wine is a learned behavior. Now after weeks or decades of doing this, as you approach your house after work and walk toward the door, without even consciously thinking about it, your brain is triggering this false need for your learned behavior—alcohol. Or perhaps you have learned to begin your weekend, Friday afternoon with a few drinks. The same applies to you.

To put it bluntly, you did this to yourself.

I did, too.

So now, you must unlearn this behavior. It won't be easy, but it's totally do-able. You will have to consciously fight the urge, the habit, for several weeks. You may be angry, frustrated, stressed, and anxious that you can't turn to this method of soothing and relaxing. I get it; I was at the beginning, too.

The sacrifice is worth it. Find the joy in the sacrifice.

The fastest way to unlearn this behavior is finding a replacement behavior. That can be in the form of a mocktail (recipes in the appendix) or filling that time when you would have had a beverage with something else: a manicure, pedicure, massage, hot bath, workout, or my favorite, shopping!

Did you know about 20 percent of the alcohol you consume is absorbed in the stomach and 80 percent in the small intestine? Now you know the liver is the main organ that processes alcohol. The liver is the largest organ you have, weighing in at a mere three pounds. Once alcohol enters your bloodstream, it remains in your body until it's fully processed. Nearly 100 percent of the alcohol is broken down by your liver; the rest is removed in your urine, breathed out by your lungs, or sweated out through your skin. Drinking too much can lead to fatty liver, which can be a dangerous diagnosis. However, all this can be reversed when you stop drinking.

Here's the most troubling point: While your liver is trying to deal with the alcohol that you've introduced, it literally stops metabolizing fats, carbs, and protein. Remember the liver's main function is to filter toxins, and when you drink, you've introduced a very large toxin, so it begins to clear it from the body. Dealing with the alcohol becomes the priority. This means that your liver will burn fat very slowly (this is what leads to fatty liver). Our bodies cannot use or store alcohol, like it does the macronutrients we have defined. So, when you drink, your body's digestive process goes on hold to deal with the alcohol.

Alcohol is empty calories.

The beer gut isn't a myth. We all "wear" our foods and alcohol. So anything (food or alcohol) that is high in simple sugars gets stored in the body as fat. For men, this is generally in their core and neck; and for ladies, this generally gets stored in the back of the legs—the hamstring area.

Yes, we wear our foods. I know you've heard we are what we eat, but the easiest way to visualize this is to point out that our foods affect every part of our body, including our skin.

Ladies, cellulite can be reversed; this should be super encouraging for you. Just remember the longer you are on one of my food plans, and avoid alcohol, the pitting in your skin will reduce along with the weight loss you experience.

Can I get an "AMEN!"

Men, the same goes for your cellulite, although you tend to have less due to the way your skin fibers are structured between skin layers. But the same can be applied to the weight you carry in your middle.

How incredible that so much of the damage we have done to our bodies can literally be reversed. Wow! Our bodies are amazing, powerful, and truly out to make us the healthiest we have ever been, if only we will do our part.

Remember, I am not saying you can never have another adult beverage. What I am saying is not now. I know you want to consistently see massive success. You won't have that the longer you try and lie to yourself that you can drink. Sweet friend, it won't happen. So what I advise my full-time clients to do is give it up, cold turkey, for twelve weeks. Then they assess the role alcohol has in their lives. Perhaps you can safely introduce a glass or two, one time a week. But the moment you see your weight loss halt, you once again must drop this behavior.

Coach Tip: Be patient with yourself. If you have long relied on alcohol to end your day, to fill your weekend, or to soothe stressful times, it will likely take three weeks to break this habit. I promise you it's worth the joyful sacrifice.

Chapter 25

The Perfect Plan

Learn to trust yourself and the process. It's easy to give up when the scale doesn't reflect your food and behavior choices. We so badly want to control the outcome. Stop! Trust the process, your intuition, and yourself.

So, what is the perfect plan?

The perfect plan is one that you will desire to execute consistently, day in, day out. The perfect plan is one that you enjoy, that doesn't cause you to starve yourself, and that makes you feel confident and stable.

The perfect plan is whatever you choose to sustain long term and will net you the results you want and deserve.

As you begin to develop and construct your plan, a word of caution: Do not start a new eating plan by immediately adding in carb cycling and intermittent fasting. It is vitally important that you systematically and purposefully introduce each strategy so that you clearly know what is working and not working for your body.

Step 1: Stabilize your metabolism. For months, years, or decades you have abused your metabolism. Our first step is to healthfully stabilize your internal fat-burning fire. The best way to do this is to choose a steady-state caloric plan that is either a 40/40/20 split of proteins, complex carbs, and healthy fats or a 40/40/20 split of protein, healthy fats, and complex carbs. I cannot stress enough that you need to pick one energy source: either complex carbs or healthy fats—NOT both—in the same meal. A steady-state caloric plan is one that has the same calories and macro breakdown every day of the week.

Once you have chosen your macronutrient split and determine which foods you will eat daily to achieve your macro goal, then give your body time to adjust to this way of eating. Allow your body time to respond to the nutrient-dense whole foods you are fueling it with. For many of you, just like many of my full-time clients, you will initially find it very difficult to eat all the food that you need. That's to be expected. You have literally been nutrient void for a long time. Your body is not used to whole, nutrient-dense foods. It's okay. However, I need you to slowly work up to all the food, all the meals on your plan. Within two to three weeks of "working up," you should be able to handle the food load that your body truly needs. If you need anything more than a three-week work up, you will need to question yourself: Are you fighting the plan and continually finding excuses not to eat? Remember, food is fuel.

I would suggest a three- to four-week phase of execution to stabilize your metabolism.

During this phase, weigh yourself once a week, not daily. Be sure to note your starting measurements (chest, smallest part of your waist, and hips) and compare measurements every other week. I have included a fantastic progress chart in the appendix for you to use. Do not expect a change in measurements weekly, but rather every two weeks. I would also advise you to take your starting pictures. I know this is difficult as no one wants to look at the hard truth, but you will regret it if you don't. Your entire physique is about to transform. Taking progress pictures weekly or every other week will play a critical role in keeping your mind on the goal.

Step 2: Overcoming plateaus. If your steady-state plan is netting you consistent weight loss, then don't alter anything. The time to consider carb cycling and/or intermittent fasting is when you feel your body has hit a weight-loss plateau. If this is the case, then choose one new strategy to implement—not both. Either choose carb cycling or intermittent fasting. Once again, allow three to four weeks to execute Step 2.

Remember, there is no wrong answer here. Carb cycling is not better or worse than intermittent fasting; they are just different. So in order to choose, I would suggest you review both chapters on the matter and then decide which strategy will better fit into your current lifestyle. Executing a 16:8 intermittent fasting protocol is not ideal for some lifestyles. Assess which will best fit into your current schedule and then execute that for the next four weeks.

NOTE: It is perfectly fine and normal to execute either intermittent fasting or carb cycling for short periods and then return to your steady-state plan.

Also note that if you are following your plan, then every three to four weeks you will want to recalculate your macros and caloric needs using the Harris-Benedict equation. If you do not recalculate, and you have been losing weight, then you will face a weight-loss plateau due to no longer being in a caloric reduced state. As you lose weight, you will need less fuel.

Coach Tip: Execute one eating style at a time. Give your body time to adjust and work for you. Rerun your calculations through the Harris-Benedict equation approximately every three to four weeks. Most of all, be consistent!

Chapter 26

Fear of Food

Can I tell you a secret? Even after losing over 100 pounds by eating a lot of food, at times I still fear food. I bet you never knew that this is a real phobia: pocrescophobia. With this phobia we often avoid food and drinks because we are scared to gain weight. But just like other phobias, this fear is irrational. But that doesn't make it any less your reality. I GET IT!

Fear of food and fear of eating can lead to eating disorders. If you feel you are suffering from an eating disorder, I want to encourage to you talk to a licensed therapist. Together, you can develop coping skills to get you to a healthier mindset. There is one marked difference between pocrescophobia and those suffering from anorexia. Those with anorexia fear the effects of food on body image. This must be addressed through cognitive behavioral therapy.

I need to help you understand that pocrescophobia leads to massive amounts of anxiety in thinking about gaining weight. When you're scared to gain weight, you may go to great lengths to avoid it, and for many that means NOT eating.

There is no clear cause of this phobia. It can develop out of weight stigmas— judging others on their weight; perfectionism (I'll raise my hand here); and the thought of "thin is ideal" and "weight gain is a flaw." Additionally, it can stem from anxiety disorders or just personal experiences.

Remember, talking to a licensed professional is incredibly helpful. We all need coping skills. So never feel embarrassed to seek out therapy.

Ninety-nine percent of the clients I help are afraid to eat. Why wouldn't we be scared? We have been told year after year that to lose weight, we have to eat less. We've also been told for decades "calories in, calories out" (meaning how much you eat versus how much you burn).

Flawed science and years of misinformation has led to billions of women starving themselves and feeling like total failures because they cannot lose weight. These same women need to fuel their body and repair their metabolism in order to shed fat.

Now, you and I both have the responsibility to unlearn everything we have been taught. While our brains want to accept the fact that we need to eat in order to lose, it's extremely difficult to have faith and believe this is true.

The thousands of clients I have coached are proof this works.

Do not fear food.

Again, I will remind you that you would never expect your car to run without gas. If you do not eat, you are expecting your body to run without fuel, and you are expecting your organs, muscles, and cells to do their jobs without the proper nutrients.

Food is not the enemy.

Your food choices, your negative experiences, and your perceived perfect look for your body are the enemy.

Your lack of proper food nutrients is the enemy.

All of my new clients say the same thing: "I cannot believe I am eating this much and losing weight." I have heard this message thousands of times. You must remember that food is fuel, and if you want your metabolism to work for you, you have to fuel it throughout the day.

I often use this analogy: If I were to ask you to build a bonfire in the morning, you would start the fire and throw on wood, kindling, and perhaps some old newspapers on it. Your metabolism is an internal fire, and for years, it's likely been out. Now you must start the fire every day. When you start the bonfire, think of that as eating breakfast. Now, throughout the day, to keep your bonfire burning, you would tend to it by adding more wood and kindling. You would stoke the fire throughout the day. In the same way, to keep your metabolic fire churning throughout the day, you need to eat. If you don't eat, the fire will go out, just as it would if you didn't tend to your bonfire. Eating several well-planned, macronutrient-balanced meals throughout the day is the best way to keep your metabolic fire churning.

So what happens if you ignore your bonfire the same way you have been ignoring the needs or your organs, muscles, and cells? The bonfire will diminish, the embers will slowly turn black, and the fire will die. The truth is, this is what you have done to your metabolic fire, by not eating enough or not eating at all.

Remember, we discussed earlier your basal metabolic rate. This is the caloric number that your body absolutely needs to survive. Many of you haven't even been eating enough to meet your basal metabolic rate. You aren't even close. When you aren't fueling your body, your body will shut down. It begins to preserve itself. This triggers your body to pull from storage—glycogen storage. This is stored energy. The metabolism then begins to slow down to preserve energy. Then your fat cells shut down and won't release fat, because you have put your body in a preservation state.

You have created a vicious cycle, all because you are choosing not to fuel your body. You are scared.

You have created your own mess, as I had, but using this book as a guide or blueprint to your lifestyle eating plan will absolutely repair the mess you have created.

You're never too old to repair your body and lose weight.

You are never too old to become stronger mentally, and to know that your past fears don't have to dictate your future.

Every time you are fearful of eating, or believe you are eating too much, remember: FOOD IS FUEL. And if you need confirmation of how much food you are eating, once again run your numbers through the Harris-Benedict equation.

Coach Tip: If at any time you feel your approach to eating food is debilitating, seek wise counsel. You need it and deserve it.

Chapter 27

Surviving and Thriving after You Fall

I'm nearly a decade into my journey, and I still fall and fail. And you know what? I'm okay with that.

You will have times, days, weeks, and even months during your journey that will fall from the "food-plan wagon".

The actual fall doesn't matter.

What does matter is:

1. What did you learn from the fall?

2. How quickly will you choose to get back on the "food-plan wagon?"

3. What coping skills can you implement now to avoid the next fall?

When most people fall off the wagon, they spend too much time and wasted emotions wallowing in guilt and shame. WHY? Because it's how we are programmed. For decades we have put food and drinks into two categories: good and bad.

Our approach toward food has been very legalistic: black and white, but no grey.

GOOD and BAD!

If we eat a food on the BAD list, WE are bad.

If we eat a food on the GOOD list, WE are good.

Even more destructive is this behavioral choice: You eat a bad food, you are filled with guilt and shame, and yet you continue to eat off-plan or continue to drink alcohol. You've now created a perpetual merry-go-round of insanity. You make the decision to continue to eat and drink off-plan because you tell yourself lies: I can't do this; I'm destined to make poor choices; I will be fat forever; this is too hard.

Well, now you're choosing to fall and stay on the ground, bleeding out.

Listen to me closely: I don't like using the word "failure," but if this is your behavior, if this is what you choose, you will absolutely fail.

You've heard this analogy before: You have one flat tire, so you decide to pop the other three.

Remember, I said you had three questions to answer:

1. What did you learn from the fall?

2. How quickly will you get back on the "food-plan wagon?"

3. What coping skills can you implement now to avoid the next fall?

As soon as you fall, you must stop and self-reflect. It should be noted that you may need to seek wise counsel on question 3.

I've mentioned my messy relationship with alcohol.

Many of my clients turn to pints of ice cream, bags and bags of Doritos, or simply NOT eating at all. All these choices can be just as destructive to our bodies.

My lesson learned when I fall with alcohol:

I use this poison to relax, to mentally unwind, to be able to breathe, and to wash away anxiety and the pit I feel in my stomach. I've learned that I personally go in cycles of working excessively. Every single time I do this, if I don't build in a forced day off, which has to include stepping outside of my house and away from the work, I will hit the invisible and quickly approaching brick wall.

How quickly will I choose to get back on the food-plan wagon?

For me, it's immediately. I don't function well off-plan. No one does.

I can literally flip a switch: off plan one day, back on plan the next. I highly recommend you do the same. Honestly, there should NOT be any other choice. The longer you sit there, ignoring your wounds from falling, ignoring the fact that you have three questions to answer to get back on plan, the more destructive you will be to your mind and body.

Once I get back on plan, do I fight temptations to drink more? Absolutely. These same temptations will happen to you, whether it's alcohol or processed or sugary foods. Withdrawal from sugar or alcohol is very real; there are well-documented stages for each. Throughout each stage is a deep chemical desire to engage with these poisons again.

Flipping the switch and immediately getting back on plan is a choice. This is your choice. Conversely, if you choose to stay off-plan longer, that's also your choice. The longer you stay down on the ground nursing your wounds, and the longer you stay off the "food-plan wagon," the more likely you are going to fail long term.

What coping skills do I now have to ensure this won't happen again?

I've willingly talked with an amazing therapist about this very subject. When I hit the brick wall, I know that there are two choices: drink or force sleep. My coping skill most of the time is to choose sleep. This is more than a small nap; this is a sleeping event. No work, no electronics. I have to force sleep for generally a full day.

Most times, I choose sleep, and I enjoy it without guilt.

However, just like you, I sometimes don't choose wisely and go for the more instant gratification: alcohol. And as you know, it never ends well. I never feel better, happier, or more confident. This choice causes more issues: guilt, self-loathing, and days of finding my confidence once again.

I should have chosen sleep.

Remember, you will fall, and when you do, you have three simple questions to answer. Don't over complicate your falls. Don't overthink the "fall." Just answer those three questions and move forward, on-plan.

Chapter 28

How Fat Escapes Your Body

I'm sure you're like me. You always want to pee and (hopefully) poop before you step on the scale. I still rejoice every time this happens in the morning. You may assume this is how fat leaves your body. NOPE!!! So buckle up while I explain the fascinating way that fat escapes your body!

You breathe it out!

Most of your fat leaves your body as carbon dioxide. Yes, some of it is expelled through sweat, tears, urine, and feces. But most fat byproducts leave your body through your breath.

Let's go one step further. It is estimated that you breathe in about 1.5 pounds of oxygen daily. This is in addition to what you eat and drink, which may add up to about 8 pounds daily. What you eat and drink needs to exit somehow if you want to lose weight. As we have discussed, your body converts fat to energy, causing the fat cells to literally shrink.

Most clients don't care how the fat escapes as long as the number on the scale goes down. But you may be curious if there is anything you can do to increase the amount of carbon dioxide you breathe out. Can you simply breathe faster? Sadly, no. I wish there were a way, because you know I'd be all over that, and you would be, too.

That said, if you are an exerciser, you may be able to increase carbon dioxide (CO_2) by performing physical activities. Clearly, swapping out an hour of lying on the couch with an hour of walking or jogging removes more CO_2 from your body and therefore improves your ability to lose weight.

Your body is working to remove CO_2 while you are sleeping as well.

Coach Tip: While none of my clients are required to exercise, because you can and will lose weight without it, here is a good case for moving your body. By the way, if you are just starting to work out, never underestimate the power of walking. Last year, I gave up jogging to preserve my aging knees, and now I power walk. It's been a fascinating experiment. I can raise my heart rate just as much through power walking as I did with running.

Section 3

Your Imperfect Journey

When I began writing this book, it was the busiest time of my career and my coaching business. Was it the perfect time, in my eyes, to start the book? No. And to top it off, we were on a very aggressive timeline. I had a few short months to complete the task.

We were serving approximately 500 clients a month, doing a complete overhaul on our website, and beginning the process of franchising our business and white-labeling all of our client deliverables.

My husband and I were swamped. For an entire month, we didn't stop working, including on the weekends. Together, we were operating on a very high-performing level.

I didn't see the brick wall coming.

After our fourth weekend of working, him coding, me writing and revising, and both of us together creating the business plan for franchising, I snapped.

Like I said, I didn't see the brick wall coming. I never do.

It was a Monday, and by noon, I was in the red zone like an angry dog. An innocent comment my husband made set me off. I couldn't recover. I needed a hard break, I needed time out of the house, and I needed to relax. By midafternoon, I had called a friend and met her for drinks.

And we drank.

A LOT!

I could feel my level of stress melt. I could literally feel myself relaxing. I could tell I was coming out of fifth gear and into first gear, and I liked that. I hadn't felt like this in a long time. In the moment, that afternoon and evening, I enjoyed drinking.

The next morning, I realized I had lost my footing and I wasn't feeling confident.

I personally have a messy relationship with alcohol. It's absolutely a love/hate relationship. For me, I'm more likely to occasionally abuse alcohol than I am food. Don't get me wrong—we all have our "thing." Everyone has a "go-to" when it comes to coping. I can go months at a time without a drink, performing at a very high level, and then the proverbial wall shows up without warning and knocks me to the ground.

Ironically, I didn't really start drinking until I married Stephen and attempted to raise seven children while working full-time and owning a CrossFit gym. And there were times when my husband would be deployed for months. The daily pressure, whether Stephen was home or not, often felt like I was a bad zit ready to be popped. In hindsight and healing, I came to recognize that I shifted my food addiction over to alcohol.

I cannot stress this enough that we all have a go-to, a "thing" that (falsely) allows us to cope. Sugar is just as bad as alcohol.

Your journey will be a very flawed—an imperfect journey. And that's okay. You simply cannot expect it to be perfect. You are not robot. There are so many outside factors to your journey, so I want you to go into this with your eyes wide open, fully knowing and expecting that you will stumble and fall.

The falls don't matter.

I've mentioned before that your mindset needs to be that you are going to execute this lifestyle plan for the rest of your life. An occasional fall won't matter in the big picture. As my dear friend Margaret says, "We aren't prepping for prom." We are in this together, for a lifetime.

When I'm sixty, I won't look back and remember this week while I was writing the book and juggling a hundred other balls in the air, when I hit the brick wall and drank. That Monday, in the big scheme of things, is a blip.

You will have many more wins, many more great days and weeks in your journey than you will have bad. Focus on the wins and not the falls. Focus on the 90 percent good and never focus on the 10 percent bad.

You are human.

You are not a robot.

Your journey will be perfectly imperfect.

But most importantly, if you work through this section, you will, once and for all, heal your relationship with food.

Chapter 29

Healthy versus Skinny

The ugly truth!

Since fourth grade, I have strived to be skinny—super lean. For three decades, this was what I longed for.

In late 2016, I competed in my first body-building competition. I weighed 146 pounds the day I stepped on stage. Remember, I'm 6 feet tall barefoot. Several weeks later, I competed in my second competition and weighed 142 pounds. I felt amazing, and frankly, I thought I looked like a Victoria's Secret model. I was wearing a size zero!

The ugly truth was that I was getting out of bed every day, taking a few steps, and falling to the ground, passing out. Even worse, several times a week I was peeing in the bed. My body was shutting down.

I had met my skinny goal, but I was far from healthy. Very far!

Everything has a purpose, and yes, getting to this extremely low weight and single-digit body fat was the intent for these competitions. I was well-conditioned, but for me, this weight was far from healthy and certainly not sustainable long term.

Before we can deep-dive into the many twists and turns you will have during your journey, and most importantly, how to handle them all, we must address whether you are striving for skinny or healthy! If you are striving for skinny, you will never truly heal your relationship with food.

The two—skinny versus healthy—are wildly different. Stop striving for skinny or thin. None of this equates to true health.

If skinny is your goal, your approach is all wrong, and your journey will be destructive to your mind and body. Skinny doesn't equal healthy; it never will. Remember, losing weight is all about lifestyle choices rather than being hyper-focused on a skinny number that you want to achieve on the scale.

If you're focusing on skinny, your choices will be extreme, and you will get lost in minor details of your meal plan. Striving for skinny will mean extreme food choices and extreme workout choices. Striving for skinny will lead to restriction and likely inconsistency. This all leads to harming your metabolism once again.

When striving for skinny, you will get lost in the details of your meal plan. One day you'll count only calories, and the next you'll count macros. You'll stop eating after 6:00 PM and therefore skip needed fuel. You'll weigh yourself all the time. Once again, you will be returning to horrible rules that you have read or false information that you've been told or heard. All this leads to confusion versus trust.

Nothing good comes from striving for skinny! Never, ever.

Friend, I'm still mentally recovering from the extremely low weight I hit when I was competing in body building (142 pounds). That season of my life was all about extremes and restrictions. I romanticize being that skinny again. Every time I beat myself up for not weighing in the 140s or even 150s, I stop that negative internal talk and remind myself of the destructive path that it was taking on my body.

For my height, a normal weight range, according to the CDC, would be from 136 to 184 pounds. That's an insanely large range. The "old" Martha would have looked at this range and thought I should be striving to weigh 136 pounds, and I would beat myself up for never getting there. Now remember, my body was shutting down in the mid-140s. I couldn't even stay warm throughout the day. No matter the outside temperature, I was literally freezing all the time. Skinny doesn't equal healthy.

If you live and die by weight and body mass index (BMI) charts, or if your doctor is comparing you to the government charts, I want you to immediately stop.

True health is not based on a number! It simply cannot be.

A lower number doesn't always equate to a healthy heart, healthy cholesterol, or healthy blood sugar, let alone a healthy mentality.

So, what does "healthy" mean to you? Sure, it could mean low blood pressure, low cholesterol, and a healthy heart. But I'm going to challenge you to define this further.

Healthy could mean:

Being able to get down on the floor with your children or grandchildren and being comfortable and able to stand back up without assistance

Being able to walk a mile without getting winded

Having clear skin

Feeling confident

Being strong enough to stay away from alcohol

Being able to sit on an airplane without a seatbelt extender

Being able to sit in a booth at a restaurant

Being able to tie your own shoes

Being able to take the steps versus an elevator

Being able to move your body without pain

Always strive for healthy! In doing so, the scale will move. Be consistent with your meal-plan routine, and at any moment when you feel like you're slipping or questioning, ask yourself this: Am I striving for skinny or healthy? Which choice should I make right now to promote being healthy?

OK, now that we have determined healthy is our goal, I want you to read the next few chapters with a very open mind. I want you to digest the truths that are coming your way. While it may not feel great to uncover exactly why you have a weight issue, the work is very important. You are about to heal your relationship with food, and in doing so, you will reveal the most BeYOUtiful version of you!

Chapter 30

Your Silent Best Friend

Through coaching thousands and thousands of clients, I now realize food (and quite often alcohol) must be viewed as a silent friend. And there are two choices for how you interact with this friend. Either you interact with food as a supportive, healthy friend, or as an abusive, destructive friend.

You're sad, you eat.

You're happy, you eat.

You want to celebrate, you eat and drink.

You're overwhelmed, you eat.

You're anxious, you eat.

You likely have never thought of this, but you have silent best friend. And this friend's name is FOOD.

Since birth, you've been both friends and enemies with FOOD.

Some days you hate food.

Some days you love food.

Some days you abuse food.

On rational days, you treat food as your best friend.

Rigid rules.

Guilt.

Binge.

This is a deeply rooted relationship you never realized you were participating in.

And now, you've entered a battle to UNDO your piss-poor relationship with food and finally heal!

Think about this: would you ever treat a best friend the way you treat your friendship with food? No, you wouldn't, as it's mildly abusive.

Your attitude toward food started at a very young age. While you were potty training, you were likely rewarded with food. If you were a good girl at the dentist, you got a lollypop. If you came home sad from school, your mother would feed you. If you got good grades, your parents would reward you with food. You see the cycle, and if you have children, you are likely repeating this cycle. Now as an adult, you can see how you are perpetuating this relationship.

Everything we celebrate is centered around food—holidays, birthdays, and anniversaries. This is how America does life. We celebrate with food. No wonder nearly 42 percent of adults are obese and another nearly 33 percent are overweight. Combine those two numbers, and over 70 percent of our society is dealing with a weight issue. Frankly, we shouldn't be surprised.

You have a silent relationship with food. For most Americans, based on these numbers, it's a horrifically poor relationship.

Right now, you are redefining your silent relationship with food. Right now, you have an opportunity to break generational habits and truly set boundaries with your friend, food. And in doing so, you will absolutely heal your relationship with food.

Step 1: The role of food in your life. Eating is defined as the consumption of food and liquid to sustain life and to meet your body's basic needs for growth, development, and function.

Notice that nowhere in the definition did it mention rewarding or comforting yourself with food. That simply isn't the role.

Step 2: Food is fuel and ONLY fuel. The foods you eat contain nutrients that provide energy (fuel) for your body to make new cells, heal, fight illness, and provide the energy you need to survive each day.

Notice again that nowhere in the definition did it mention rewarding or comforting yourself with food. Again, it's not the role.

The reality is that we've abused food and put it into a role for which it was never intended.

The moment you can recognize and believe that food is merely fuel is when you will begin to redefine the role food has in your life. Time after time, as you go to grab the wine or ice cream or order pizza, you simply need to repeat: Food is ONLY fuel.

Food will never solve the emotional issues spinning in your life; food will never fix a broken marriage; food will never fill the hole in your heart; food will never repair a broken relationship with a sibling or parent.

Now listen closely, because this next statement is vitally important:

> **Food didn't cause the weight issue. Your weight issue is the by-product of all the emotional crap in your life—perhaps decades long, or for some, it just started recently. Food is the symptom of all the junk you have endured.**

Think of it this way: you are an iceberg. The weight issue is the tip of the iceberg, the visible part. But the iceberg, like your weight issue, developed from what lies beneath the water.

Food will never solve the iceberg in your life! Stop expecting it to.

Food is merely fuel for your body, and that's IT!

Chapter 31

The Iceberg

For one year, I coached an incredible woman who lost 72 pounds. She looked amazing, nearly unrecognizable by those who knew her at her heaviest. Personally, I was shocked and amazed at how she diligently worked her plan and how her skin responded to her drastic weight loss. She rushed to what she thought was the finish line. Then, slowly, she returned to her old way of eating. Very slowly, the weight crept back on. She, like many others, had lost her footing.

I have seen this time after time. Clients rush to the finish line with blinders on, and then they stumble and never regain their footing. Here is why:

You have a weight issue, but that's only the tip of the iceberg.

Everyone can see the tip of the iceberg. You can see it for miles. It's bright and shiny and looks massive. But we all know that what's under the surface of the water is larger and stronger. It's massive.

Your weight issue is the tip of the iceberg. Literally.

It's what you can see in the mirror.

You see it in your clothes. You see the inflammation in your face, belly, arms, fingers, and legs. You see the fat.

As for the iceberg, what you don't see is the massive structure beneath the water, the destructive mass that has ripped mighty ships into pieces. But what's below the surface is what constitutes a danger.

Back to your weight issue and your personal tip of the iceberg: Your visible weight issue has likely been caused by everything lurking below the water, which for you could be one or many events, emotions, false perceptions, and lies you believe.

Maybe for you, "under the water" is:

Emotional abuse.

Physical abuse.

Decades of rejection by the opposite sex.

A poor parent-to-child relationship.

A failed marriage.

A difficult teenage child.

Being fired from a job.

Being raped or molested.

A scary health diagnosis.

The death of a parent, sibling, or close friend.

All this and much, much more creates your massive personal iceberg—your weight issue.

I can't tell you what is below your surface. Only you can explore, discover, and define what led to your personal tip of the iceberg. What I can tell you is that now is the time to face these emotions head on. For if you don't, you will continue to lose weight, gain weight, lose weight, and gain weight again. You will never get off the weight-loss rollercoaster because you haven't addressed the real issue(s) that led to you gaining weight. You will never heal your relationship with food!

For me, my iceberg grew slowly, and it formed because I didn't get the attention from the opposite sex that I thought I needed. It formed because I have an obsessive desire for unrealistic perfection. It grew wildly out of rejection from my first husband.

The formation of your iceberg doesn't have to be from a traumatic event. In fact, it can slowly grow from a series of small choices, things people have said to you, and decisions you have made.

The base of your personal iceberg has energy, and that very energy is overtaking your life. It's manifesting into your weight issue, and until you dig into the reasons WHY you have your weight issue, you will not have massive, long-term success. And you will perpetually diet.

You can and will lose weight, but along this journey, you MUST face the issues that caused you to get here, the part of the iceberg that lies beneath the water. Because if you ignore that, you will gain all the weight back and likely more. The core issues must be addressed.

Chapter 32

What Lies Beneath the Water

My first memory of thinking I was fat was in fourth grade. The entire class was about to leave for recess. I stood by the classroom door, and behind me was a boy named Brian and several other boys. I don't remember what led up to him saying this, but he called me "Big Bertha"!

I was devastated, of course.

I don't remember anything else from that school day until I got home and was bawling in front of my parents. I remember exactly where I was standing: in our family room, which was now my parent's office, as my father owned his own CPA practice. He and my mother worked together on the business. Our family room was full of desks—my father's, my mother's, and three others, one for each daughter to do homework. Mine was on the end.

I was leaning against my desk, still in my school clothes, tears running from my eyes. My father stood in front of me. I recounted the story and how Brian called me that horrible name. My father, standing strong and mighty at 6 foot 8 inches, said this to me: "Marth, it could be worse. At least you have two arms."

My father, Tom, had lived his own battles.

At the age of ten, he fell from a ladder and broke his right arm. With his elbow exposed, his mother, Anna, rushed him to the emergency room. The intern never fully cleaned or set his arm properly before casting it. Within days, my father had a fever and landed back in the hospital nearing death from gas gangrene.

Gas gangrene is a bacterial infection that develops from an injury or a surgical wound that's depleted of blood supply. It's fast-spreading and life threatening.

The infection had spread quickly. My father was going to die.

The only way to save Tommy, as he was called as a child in the mid-1940s, was to operate and amputate.

The Philadelphia hospital wanted to get "ahead" of the infection. But it was too late. They amputated his right arm as high as they could, nearing the shoulder. Sadly, the infection had spread through his entire body. He was dying, and the doctors weren't sure what to do.

Penicillin had just been invented. It didn't work.

Then a Chicago doctor, flown in by the hospital as they feared a massive liability case, suggested a very experimental treatment—expose Tommy's body to pure oxygen via a contraption the doctors called a "steel lung."

I vaguely remember my father telling this story to many people. He was put in a "steel lung" and breathed pure oxygen. These treatments went on for weeks, multiple times a day. The goal was to steadily increase the amount of oxygen in his blood to kill off the gas gangrene.

My father was in the hospital over a month. He celebrated his eleventh birthday there. And he finally left, very weak, without his right arm—the very arm with which he learned to write and play the piano.

His mother, Anna, a short and rigid German woman, showed no mercy. She pushed my father to be self-reliant and self-sufficient. She also demanded that he continue to study piano, but now, with only one hand, his non-dominant hand.

He learned to dress, tie his shoes, tie a tie, and even play baseball with one arm.

No one was coming to save Tommy. No one was coming to do it for him.

Only he was responsible for turning his pain into progress.

So yes, my father had his own battles, and as an adult I can see why I didn't get the empathy I needed as a young girl on that defining day.

That day, when I clearly needed reassuring words from the man I loved the most, I didn't get it.

And that's OK! I do not harbor bad feelings for my father. He did HIS best.

Was it ideal? No, of course not.

But it started to build me into the strong, self-reliant, self-sufficient woman I am today. However, when Brian called me "Big Bertha," a seed was planted in my heart, and that seed grew and grew, like a wild weed! I allowed it to grow; I was manifesting that label. And when I didn't get the reassurance from the father I loved, sadly, that seed got watered, and there was no killing it.

My father was correct—at least I had two arms—but what many don't realize is that while physical scars like my father's are so easy to see, emotional scars hurt just as bad.

Throughout middle school and high school, I continued to carry "Big Bertha" with me every day. When I was on a diet, I was a good girl, and therefore Big Bertha was quieted. When I wasn't on a diet, I was a bad girl and living out my calling of being Big Bertha. Daily, I was manifesting Big Bertha.

Into my teens and early twenties, I just wanted to be recognized for more than my brain and abilities. Anything I chose to pursue, I excelled at. But the one thing I was longing for was for someone to recognize me for my beauty, not my abilities. I just wanted a boy/man to think I was beautiful.

We always want what we don't have.

This unhealthy but very deep desire would grow, quietly and deeply like an iceberg, well into my thirties and through my first marriage.

For decades, I didn't get that attention, so I continued to turn to food. Food filled the hole in my soul, or so I thought.

What I didn't see or even realize was I was slowly creating my iceberg.

During your journey, you will have to be brave. You will have to admit your role in your weight issue. You will have to talk about how others contributed to your issue as well. Remember, this is your story, your reality, and no one can tell you otherwise. Your perception of how you got to where you are is your reality.

I have challenged my full-time clients to address their own icebergs that led to their weight issues, and when they do, the stories they tell are gut-wrenching. I've heard stories of rape, name-calling, abusive husbands, deep depression, and sibling jealousy and hatred. There is always a common thread, whether it was a traumatic event in childhood (yes, name-calling can be traumatic for a young child) or event(s) in adulthood, these moments lead to all of us turning to food as a protective shelter and emotional comfort.

You are poised to live a life of purpose and confidence in your imperfect journey, but I cannot stress enough that if you ignore the events and emotions that created your personal iceberg, you will likely gain the weight back. If you ignore this step, you are ignoring the most important piece of your journey: self-discovery. Healing and food addictions can be broken, but it will require you to be honest about what got you to this point.

Chapter 33

Turning Pain into Progress or Own Your Mess

I shared in a national television interview that for decades, I felt unlovable—not by God, but by man.

Looking back and exposing why I felt this way seems ridiculous. But a series of small events and choices all added up to this horrible feeling:

Being called Big Bertha.

Being put on a diet as a child, even though I was not overweight.

Having an adult neighbor tell me I looked much better in pictures than I looked in person.

Not having a boyfriend in high school when it seemed everyone else did.

Having to ask a boy to my junior prom.

Not having a date for my senior prom.

Not having a boyfriend in college when it seemed every other girl around me did.

Being called horrible names, behind my back, by a college roommate.

Falling into my first marriage to a man who wanted his wife to look like anyone but me and projected his own weight issues on me.

All of this added up, in my head, to feeling that I wasn't thin enough or pretty enough, that I didn't have big enough boobs or skinny enough legs, and that I was too tall. These thoughts—plus being on a diet since age nine; and comments along the way from boys, men, and relatives—are what created my personal iceberg and contributed to a perpetual weight issue.

Once my first marriage ended, I noticed other men around me, noticing me. Very honestly, this is when I started to heal. Tall, successful men were paying attention to me. I suddenly thought maybe I wasn't ugly. Maybe I was lovable.

The real healing, however, occurred with Stephen, my second and forever husband. No, this didn't happen overnight; healing takes time. Wounds are deep, and my personal iceberg was (and frankly, still is) large. There was a lot under the water to reveal and heal. But Stephen, since day one, always reminded me that confidence is sexy, and apparently, I ooze it on the surface. I found safety in revealing my iceberg to Stephen. At times, I continue to see my therapist to talk through even more of my healing. Like I said, it will not be an overnight process, but dear friend, it's totally worth it.

So what lies beneath the water of your personal iceberg? Can you start to identify this?

Exposing the pain—what lies beneath the water—leaves you feeling raw!

You may not have any idea how to tackle or process the exposed pain. I would be remiss if I didn't mention that you, like me, may need to seek wise counsel. This is more than a girlfriend, parent, or spouse. Talking to a licensed counselor or therapist is healthy and nothing to be ashamed of.

This person will give you the coping skills you need, a clear direction, and a mental and emotional path to process the exposed pain.

With the pain exposed, you have an opportunity to own your mess and to turn your pain into progress. Through this, healing will occur!

When you own your mess, you will experience freedom, and in this case, freedom from food!

I urge you to see this as an opportunity. A window has opened, and you must walk through it to get through it.

No one is perfect.

Don't accept defeat.

Shut out negativity.

Focus forward.

Take small baby steps.

Drop any excuses.

Become self-aware.

My mother was a grade-school teacher in Delaware County, Pennsylvania. I remember her telling me this story of a young boy who lived on our street and played daily with my middle sister, Cathy. He knew my mother personally, and in her classroom, he would talk incessantly and get out of his chair, obviously causing issues. Clearly, he felt too comfortable with my mother outside of school, and his young brain couldn't adapt to the teacher/student boundary they needed in the classroom.

My mother warned young Johnny time after time that he had to stop interrupting the class with his chatter and getting out of his seat. Johnny didn't listen. Nothing would stop the boy. So my mother took matters into her own hands. She literally duct taped the boy to his chair.

This story cracks me up for two reasons. First, that my mother duct taped Johnny to his chair, and second, that she could. Hello, 1960s.

Here's why I tell you this story. You have all the control you need over your life. You may not feel that you do, but sweet friend, YOU DO. You aren't duct taped to the "chair" of life. You are never trapped. You are never stuck. You are never doomed to a miserable life.

You may feel that you are. But that's a lie you are choosing to believe.

Rip off the duct tape. This means exposing what lies beneath your iceberg.

Then stand up and believe healing is coming your way!

Seek wise counsel. Own your mess. And now the healing will begin!

Turn your pain into incredible progress, and own your mess!

PS: Even when Johnny was duct taped to the chair, he continued to get up and walk the classroom with the chair taped to him.

PPS: Be like Johnny.

Chapter 34

Under Attack

You are in a fight against your biggest opponent—you. Your fears, doubts, and insecurities are searching for a weak spot, a crack in your armor. This is war, so prepare your mind and heart for battle.

Have you ever noticed that every time you start something incredibly important, something you know will propel you to a higher level in your life, you soon feel under attack? If you're a believer, you will recognize that Satan seems to attack when he thinks it's to his advantage. None of this is accidental. When the devil perceives that your work will further the Kingdom of God or you are prepped for a great breakthrough, he will attack.

Whether you believe in spiritual attacks or feel like the universe is against you, the premise is the same.

Listen to me: You are prepped to win, but it will take perseverance. You may be thinking, "This isn't the right time." No, that is not the case; in fact, it's quite the opposite. You are on the brink of a breakthrough in your life. The path is never easy, but if you go into this battle with your weight, you will have to push through fear, negative thoughts, hopeless feelings, and the desire to quit.

If you feel that the mental warfare you are going through is like hell, push through and keep going. You must go through it to get through it.

No, you are not destined to be at your current weight forever. No, you are not destined to be "stuck" in your current body.

Your timing to begin the weight-loss battle is not wrong. Believe that 100 percent. This is not the time to quit, nor is this the time to fail to launch. No one said this was easy. If it were easy, we wouldn't have an obesity pandemic in America.

You already made the decision to be the minority and not eat like the majority of Americans. Stand up—there is a breakthrough staring you in the face, but you must stand strong, push through fears and opposition, and battle on.

The ironic part of all this is that the attacks are often disguised via your spouse, significant other, friends, and even your job. Many of my clients come to me in distress due to a spouse trying to continually sabotage them not only with off-plan foods, but also with non-supportive words. Or their friends express ugliness as they lose weight. (We'll cover this shortly.) These sabotaging actions and words truly don't matter. However, you need to realize your journey has suddenly made many around you feel uncomfortable. You have embarked on something they only wish they could conquer. You are on your own journey, and you aren't responsible for how others feel or react to it.

I bet you're thinking I sound extremely cold-hearted right now. I am not being dismissive of other's thoughts or feelings. But this book is not about them—it is meant to guide you to the most authentic, beYOUtiful, and glorious life you could live on Earth. Hopefully, by setting an amazing example for those around you, they will join you in their own time. So remember, sweet friend, there will be attacks, many battles, and opposition from others. You are not responsible for making them comfortable with your journey.

Stand up, solider. This battle is yours. It's you versus you.

Expect the attacks. Push through to a better you.

And my greatest word of advice? Breathe.

Then laugh at the attacks, because you are stronger than anything pushed your way. The devil will never win! You have power over him. You are a child of God!

In the upcoming chapters, we'll discuss goal setting, which will also set you up to battle through the attacks.

Now I want you to realize some of the push-back for your journey is something I call the "mirror syndrome," which I'll explain in depth in the next chapter.

Chapter 35

The Mirror Syndrome

Remember when I told you that when I was divorcing my first husband, I had "friends" in my church who "sprayed me with the Christian can of Lysol"? My divorce was making them very uncomfortable, so they were angry with me and abandoned me without ever really understanding my point of view concerning my failing marriage.

The same scenario, different friends, occurred as I pushed to lose the last forty pounds and began my journey into bodybuilding. Everything I was doing was making those around me feel very uncomfortable. I could recognize it this go-around, because I had been down this path before, a decade earlier. So this time, there weren't any feelings of hurt; I knew what was happening. I recognized the "mirror syndrome" and realized that the rejection occurring this time was simply revealing the character of those "friends."

You, too, will have to face the mirror syndrome. Sweet friend, it will hurt. Your success is a mirror to their failure!

The mirror syndrome is simply this: You are a mirror to someone else. Others see in you something they feel they either cannot do or have tried and failed to do, so they look at you and perhaps are jealous or angry with you. Or perhaps your new healthy choices for food means they no longer have approval or an enabler on their side, so their poor choices of food make them feel incredibly uncomfortable.

You are implementing and executing something they only wish they could. You are succeeding. You are eating unlike they are. You are no longer enabling their bad habits. You are choosing success, and in turn, you are saying no to their unhealthy events. You are saying no to always celebrating with food. You are choosing health, and this is making those around you very uncomfortable.

Their feelings of fear, anger, or jealousy will manifest very interestingly. Keep your eyes wide open. Show these people grace, but do not sacrifice your journey for their comfort zone.

Here is the most important advice: Don't take this personally. Outside relationships generally mirror the relationship we have with ourselves. So follow me here: If you are trying to better yourself and push yourself out of a comfort zone, which includes food and alcohol crutches, that means you are pushing yourself into a new level of life. Your current circle of friends—and dare I say, some marriages—may not be able to rise to this new level with you.

Yikes, that's scary, right?

You are pushing to love your innermost being and beYOUtiful. For years, even decades, your relationship with you may have been incredibly destructive, so you likely attracted people around you who innately were also somewhat destructive. But you're breaking from these destructive behaviors and choices right now, and you are starting to heal!

This is the point where communication, compromise (but not a compromise of your health, happiness, and fulfillment), and conflict resolution become vitally important. This may also be the point where you lose the friends you're meant to lose. You will either grow together or fall apart.

So how can you survive this phase?

This is the moment where everyone involved must own their mess. You've already stepped up and owned your personal mess if you've begun your food plan. You are striving daily for true health, and you are setting a strong example to those around you. Now those who are projecting fear, manipulation, and anger need to own their mess. Only then can you redefine your relationship. You cannot do this alone, and conflict cannot continue while you pursue your journey.

Be consistent with your actions. Do not break your food plan for your saboteur. You are on a journey they likely will not understand or are too fearful to begin, let alone continually execute! Their actions or reactions may or may not be intentional, so recognize the negative social event and plan for the next time this arises, because it will arise again.

There are always solutions, if you seek them out.

Here are a few scenarios and solutions:

Your mother shows up with your favorite dessert!

Deep breath. Remember, your mother grew up and likely raised you to believe that we reward others with food, and we show our love to others with food. All you need to do is thank her and remind your sweet mother than you're on this amazing journey for true health. Point out to her how you're feeling on this journey. Offer her a piece of the dessert and move on. You don't need to indulge, and if she is making you feel guilty, remind her that you love the gesture, but for you, now is not the time to partake.

If she leaves the dessert for you to eat later, throw it away.

Your family refuses to eat the new, healthier versions of meals you are cooking!

First, don't change things overnight for the entire family—unless they are on board, of course. Take it slowly for your family. Now, by no means am I saying you have to make two different meals and become everyone's personal chef. Instead, for example, prepare plain chicken, and you have your approved, non-sugary, low-fat sauce that you can add on top for yourself, while they pour ketchup or barbeque sauce on theirs.

As you introduce foods for your family, remind them how important your journey is and that it was cooked with love and with their health in mind as well. Remind them how these foods will help them feel full of energy and it will also improve their lives.

Don't forget the recipes I have included here as well, and you will likely want to access our recipe website, also discussed in the appendix of this book. Trust me, when they taste the remastered recipes that we offer, they will fall in love with this way of eating.

Your best friend wants to take you out for drinks and appetizers!

This is a tough one; we all crave girl time! Thank her and then suggest that you go shopping together or perhaps get a manicure and pedicure. Find a replacement "event" that will still allow you to be together and share a few hours together. (We discuss more of this in the next chapter.)

Remember, few will support or even take the time to understand the journey you are on. That's okay—their approval or encouragement is not needed. This is solely for you, and only you can execute this. The reward of the journey will be beyond amazing!!

Your journey is yours alone. Never expect anyone around you to understand, accept, or appreciate your journey. Yes, you will likely lose the friends that you were meant to lose, but I promise you, you will find strong, like-minded new friends who will bring you even greater joy than you could ever imagine.

Chapter 36

Discovering Replacement Behaviors

Soon after I married Stephen, we agreed he could take a deployment over to Iraq. He was gone for only four months, but those were four very long months. I was a new full-time mom to his four children and was raising my own three young children. It was horribly intense, and quite frankly, I wasn't enjoying any of it. It was too much. It was summer. I was working full time, we had a part-time nanny at home, and things weren't going well at all. I received calls almost daily from the nanny with issues at home surrounding the kids—their behavior, lack of respect, and daily antics. Many times, I would have to leave work and head home to deal with multiple issues. Frankly, I was embarrassed and was hating my life.

Blended families are a tough business. I had seven children under the age of fourteen, and Stephen's children were once again dealing with their father who was deployed. Their biological mother wasn't in the picture. It was seven kids versus one adult, and I was failing.

To be honest, I never really started to drink until I married Stephen. As I've mentioned earlier in the book, while Stephen was deployed, my dinners consisted of alcohol with sleeping pills for dessert. Or I would pile all seven kids in the SUV and head to the nearest Mexican restaurant for a pile of chips, cheese sauce, guacamole, and of course, several margaritas. This was how I coped and relaxed! Once again, I was turning to food to fill a serious void.

Doing this repeatedly created many learned behaviors. Coping with seven children, without any support, meant alcohol with a side of Mexican food, became my silent best friend. Even when Stephen returned, the learned behavior continued. All of these events led to my highest weight ever and then, ultimately, my becoming undone. But it also led to this amazing, life-changing beYOUtiful journey.

The only way to undo a learned behavior like this is to find and implement replacement behaviors. There was no way, after months and months (maybe years) of learning to cope with alcohol while raising seven kids, would I be able to go cold-turkey and be successful. I had shifted my food addiction to alcohol.

Whatever your learned behavior is, you can find a way to replace that with something that is in line with your health journey. The simplest way to approach this is finding a new behavior choice that will replace the unwanted target behavior.

Teachers use this cognitive behavior method with young children. For example, if a student continues to blurt out, he is taught to eliminate the blurting by raising his hand and waiting to be called upon. I'm not sure my mother's approach to duct taping Johnny to the chair was a valid replacement behavior, but at least we can have a good laugh about that.

So now it's your turn to identify which learned behaviors you have in your life that need a simple replacement. A word of caution: You will have to fight through the urge to return to your destructive, learned behavior. This isn't like flipping a switch. Choosing the replacement behavior will take time to adjust to. Of course, at first it won't be nearly as "satisfying" as junk food or alcohol. What I can promise you is that soon the replacement behavior will be second nature. The pride you will have for avoiding food or alcohol for emotional comfort will be much greater than actually wanting the crappy food or alcohol!

Chapter 37

Believing in Your Journey: Visualization to Manifestation

In the summer of 2016, I weighed 180 pounds, which is a healthy weight for my tall six-foot frame. I was happy, but honestly, I felt there was something more. On a whim, I decided to change my workout structure from CrossFit to that of a bodybuilder. I told my new trainer I had no desire to compete, but I wanted to change the look of my physique a bit. Famous last words.

Within a few weeks, I had committed to competing, but to do so, I entered a twenty-two-week competition prep season. Brutal. During those twenty-two weeks, I didn't have one alcoholic drink, I ate six meals a day, and I never cheated. I did five split-body part strength workouts a week, and I averaged 220 minutes of running a week.

I was a machine. I had blinders on. Nothing was going to stop me.

beyoutiful

The weight fell off me. Slowly, my food for fuel would be reduced, and as any body builder will tell you, the sport is all about manipulating food. Leading into the competition, I was in starvation mode.

During the twenty-two weeks, I would visualize my popping abs and chiseled legs. I would visualize what I wanted my body to look like.

I would lie in bed and visualize myself on stage, performing my routine and poses. I would visualize the lights following me graciously walking across the stage in five-inch heels, nearly naked, in a competition suit. I believed wholeheartedly in the end of this phase of my journey.

If you think you, you can.

If you think you can't, you can't and won't.

Visualization is a subtle shift in your mindset, and even better, it is a free tool for your weight loss. You can visualize your ideal body! Are you lean, muscular, fit, toned? What size do you wear? What kinds of clothes are you wearing at your smaller size? What kinds of foods are you eating to manifest your visualization? Visualize yourself walking into rooms and owning them. Visualize yourself proud of you. Visualize people complimenting you or your spouse acknowledging your hard work. Visualize yourself walking into any clothing store and picking any types of clothes and they will fit.

All these forward-thinking, positive images and thoughts are now burnt into your subconscious mind. And, in turn, your mind will direct your actions. Just as you clearly know your negative self-talk affects your psyche, the opposite—positive body thoughts and visualization—will positively affect your journey and the emotions you experience. Every thought you have either negatively or positively affects your brain and therefore your actions.

Not once did I ever visualize falling on stage or forgetting a pose. Even writing that sounds ridiculous, but you get my point. I believed in the end of this phase of my journey!

Visualization requires you to abandon worries, doubts, and other negative thoughts and fears. Those thoughts do not allow you to manifest your visualization. They will only halt your progress, and even worse, lead to self-sabotaging.

You know that having victory over weight loss is just as much, if not more, a mental game than it is the foods you eat. Remember, if you think you can, you can; and if you think you can't, you can't and won't. The choice is all yours.

When my first marriage ended, I took time to write out exactly what I wanted in my next partner. I was no longer going to settle, and I wanted to push through to find what I thought would be the best mate for me.

I remember making a list of thirteen attributes:

He had to be 6 foot 5 or taller

He had to make $100,000 or more

He had to be a Type A personality

He needed to be a great communicator

He had to be driven, but have deep emotions and be able to talk through his emotions

He had to understand that I was fiercely independent and strong-willed, and he had to know how to deal with me (because I'm a lot, my friend)

He had to believe in God

The list went on and on. I typed this on my laptop and saved it to my desktop, and frankly, I forgot about it. I went on many, many dates and had a few short-term relationships before I met Stephen, my husband.

A few weeks into dating him, I remembered I had typed my list. That night, I opened the file on my laptop and read it again.

I was astonished. Every single point on my list described Stephen exactly. Within four weeks, we were engaged, and nine months later we married.

No, that list has not made our marriage perfect. But I can tell you this, there is no other person on this Earth who can meet my needs and be able to handle my personality. That simple list set me up for a solid foundation of what I knew I needed to thrive in my next marriage.

I have provided you with a solid blueprint to success and meal plans in this book!! But this book won't make you successful. It provides you with a foundation of success and ways to heal your relationship with food! You still must do the work, just as I must continually work together with Stephen on our marriage.

Making my list was my way believing in a different outcome to my journey, visualizing and then manifesting Stephen. Yes, of course, I believe God had his hand in this as well, but prepping this list of wants and needs set me up for success. It defined what I wanted and needed, and I knew I wouldn't settle until I found him.

Whether you have just started your meal plan or are returning to this chapter later in your journey, you must believe in the endgame, the end of your journey. Now, let me be clear: When you're on a wellness journey, you are never really done or hit a finish line, but along the way as you set goals to meet (discussed in the next chapter), you have to believe in that goal; that end-point.

Chapter 38

Goal Setting

When I first started my wellness journey in 2012, at the age of 40, my goal was to weigh 200 pounds. That seemed reasonable for my tall six-foot body. Within ten months, I had lost a little over fifty pounds, and my goal was met. I honestly thought I was done. As you know, that wasn't the finish line. Frankly, the finish line doesn't exist when you're on a wellness journey. We'll soon deep dive into what maintenance looks like.

Goal setting. Whether you are in the first or three hundredth week of your journey, goal setting must be established. There are months when I don't take the time to set a goal and then break it into weeks, and when I don't take the time to do so, my maintenance suffers. The same will apply to your weight-loss journey.

Goal setting doesn't have to take hours, and frankly, I make it quite simple for our full-time clients. For your reference, I have dropped a goal setting sheet in the appendix for you to use each month.

There are two goal-setting categories you need to establish:

ADDITION

ELIMINATION

If you focus on these two categories, you will easily establish your monthly goals. So let's break this out.

Rule #1: Do not focus on the number of pounds or the number on the scale that you would like to reach this month or week. If you do focus on this, you will set yourself up for disappointment. Remember your body is super complex, and setting a scale goal will have you become hyper-focused on a number. Plus, a weight-loss journey is never a linear, downward process.

Rule #2: Focus ONLY on your choices and behaviors when goal setting.

Let's break this out!

Addition = What do you commit to adding to your schedule to achieve your weight goal this month? For example: Will you commit to adding weekly food preparation? Will you commit to adding in additional water? Will you commit to adding in some movement for your body?

Notice that nowhere in my ADDITION goals have I mentioned the scale or inches lost.

Elimination = What are willing to eliminate this month to achieve your weight-loss goal? For example: Will you fully eliminate alcohol for one month? Will you eliminate a social event that you clearly know will have you fall off-plan? Will you eliminate negative self-talk for 30 days?

Again, notice that there is no mention of the scale or measurements.

If you can define two or three additions and eliminations, then allow those additions and eliminations to be your behavioral guide. In turn, you will lose weight. Each addition and elimination goal will change and alter your current behaviors and choices to align with your weight-loss goal.

Once you have established your addition and elimination goals for the month, it's easy to break this out by week, if you need to. For example, I have clients who set "miles walked" goals for each month. Once they know the monthly mileage, they can easily determine their weekly goal. Then on a Sunday evening or Monday morning, they review their weekly goal and attack it.

Every Wednesday, I take just a few minutes to do a self-check-in, and I would strongly suggest you do the same. Where are you with your weekly goal, and how are you feeling about your behaviors and choices? Wednesdays are a great time to focus forward to your weekend. What challenges do you know are already planned for your weekend? Look ahead and plan. Friday or Saturday mornings are a time where I like to celebrate what I've done that week. One of these mornings I take my weekly progress pictures. Inevitably, if I have executed my addition and elimination goals, then I will see progress.

Remember, behaviors and choices will always trump the number on the scale. If you focus on behaviors and choices, the scale will reflect a loss. Solely focusing on the scale will lead to disappointing yourself, questioning yourself, questioning your plan, and at times paving a path for self-sabotage.

Do not over-complicate your monthly goals. I never want you to feel overwhelmed by the enormity of your journey. Thirty days will fly by, I promise you, and you will be amazed at how easy it is each month to define a few simple goals.

Chapter 39

Maintenance

No one warned me. When I lost over 100 pounds, I truly thought it would just "stick" and I'd be fine. I honestly thought my body would allow me to maintain the 150-pound range. But our bodies are much more complicated, and they fight us for the first year, or more, after we have lost weight.

Yes! Your body will fight you. Whether you lost ten pounds or two hundred pounds, your body will fight you for about a year. Your body is defending the old you, the higher weight, a more "comfortable" range. You are not alone; this happens to everyone.

For many, maintaining their weight isn't very motivating. This is the biggest issue. As you lose weight, you are excited to see the changes in your body, you are thrilled to buy smaller clothes, and you love seeing the scale progress downward. In maintenance, you have none of this. You're wearing the same size clothing, you watch your weight vary in a "safe window" of about five to seven pounds, and the physical transformation is complete. Where's the fun? Where is the excitement? Where is the celebration when you no longer have these incredible markers of success? The compliments stop. Your friends and family have accepted the new you, the smaller you, and the praise of your progress ceases. The attention is no longer on you and your incredible journey. Sounds depressing, right?

Don't worry, you will survive this stage, but the motivation will have to be internal. Now is the perfect time to really define the NEW YOU, but we'll cover that in upcoming chapters.

How do you maintain?

Ready?

You just never stop.

Yes, I know that is over-simplified, but it's the truth. I've said this many, many times with the hope that it will truly sink in: Your wellness journey is never over. To some extent, you will always be working some type of food plan. Do not be discouraged by this. Remember the "old you" didn't use a food plan, and where did that get you? Or think of it this way—you never stop saving for your retirement, but you are continually working some type of savings plan. The same should be true for you to maintain true health. Will you need to be "legalistic" about your plan? Likely not, unless you have a week or so that is off-plan and you need structure to lose a few pounds and get back to a comfortable maintenance weight.

Let's break this out. What does a maintenance food plan look like? And can you regularly incorporate treat meals?

Remember in the beginning of the book we identified your basal metabolic rate and your total daily expenditure? We will once again need to calculate these numbers based on your lower weight. Once again, you should refer to the Harris-Benedict equation, but this time, you will run your maintenance numbers.

Let's calculate an example client:

Female Client age 49

Height: 6 feet

New weight: 170 pounds

Activity: desk job, but works out three to four times a week

NOTE: Remember the Harris-Benedict equation is just that—a number—and doesn't calculate health or hormone issues. Use this number as a reference.

Let's do a quick review: Your basal metabolic number is the number of calories you need to survive.

Your total energy expenditure is the average number of calories you burn per day.

Many weight loss coaches would tell you, for maintenance, you need to eat the average number of calories you burn each day (your total energy expenditure). I personally like to approach this differently.

Remember in Section 1 of the book, I also introduced you to a simple equation to calculate your calorie deficit? I told you to take your starting weight, multiply that number by 10, and then subtract 10 to 15 percent. This gave you the number of calories you needed to eat to lose weight.

So let's reverse this equation. We'll use the example client above. Her new, low weight is 170 pounds. We will multiply that number by 10 (1,700) and then ADD 10 to 15 percent, and that is her new caloric range for maintenance. This means our example client will eat between 1,870 and 1,955 calories a day to maintain her weight.

Once you know the caloric range for maintenance, you can easily calculate your macronutrient split. Remember, it can be a 40/40/20 split of lean protein, complex carbs, and healthy fats, or you can reverse the energy source and have a higher healthy fat percentage and lower complex carb percentage. Now that you are in maintenance, you know which energy source is better for your unique body.

Let me give you an example of what I do:

First, I execute a 16:9 intermittent fasting protocol daily. Generally, once a week, I will execute a twenty-four-hour fast. But remember, any time you consider such a fast, it must have purpose. Never use a twenty-four-hour fast just because it sounds fun or interesting or for punishment for overeating. There should be reasons for it. For me, it's to drop a small amount of weight (perhaps a few ounces), and for a few days I haven't been hungry.

This will temporarily shock my body and bring back my hunger and the desire for food as fuel. Most days, I log all my food (still) in My Fitness Pal to ensure that I truly am hitting my macro and calorie goals. I am no longer legalistic about the food plan, and I trust that throughout the entire week, I will consistently meet my goals.

For many of my maintenance clients, they enjoy a planned treat meal about every two weeks. You can expect to do this as well. Have fun with the treat meal, but remember to reference the guidelines we outlined about treat meals. Personally, I don't have a desire to have a treat meal every week or every other week. I like to plan something special with my husband, and that usually occurs once a month.

Here is what's most important: If you are having too many treat meals, you will begin to feel less confident, you will begin to internally question WHO you are, and yes, the weight will creep back on. Only you can determine the timing and amount of treats you have. But if you feel as if you have lost that internal peace, then back off. If you realize that your old habits have started to emerge again, back off the treat meals. Step back and assess if you have begun anew or reverted to an old learned behavior that needs to be addressed.

Maintenance is about riding a wave. Some days you're on top of the wave and in full control. Some days you are in the middle of the wave as it's about to crest, and some days you're hitting the shore. This is life. DO NOT expect maintenance to be easy or simple. You must learn to ride the wave. And if at any time you have packed on a few pounds, immediately revert to your last weight loss plan and execute! This is exactly what I do as well.

You are never a failure or doomed if you gain some weight. Remember, life is complicated, and stressors are never expected or planned. Just make sure you are not consistently reverting to the OLD you and old learned behaviors.

At the start of this chapter, I mentioned that your body will fight you. Your body has a comfortable spot (weight-wise) and it will want to return to that number. That number is generally when you had a bit more stored fat than perhaps you do at your lowest weight. This fight is normal and should be expected.

I have a client named Julie. She showed amazing progress in less than a year, losing over 80 pounds. At the beginning, she weighed 242 pounds, and she reached a low of 153 pounds. Very honestly, at her lowest weight, she appeared too skinny for her five-foot, eleven-inch frame. She was a machine on a mission, and she was incredibly legalistic with her weight-loss plans that she received from me. Over the last year, she and I have been working together as her body fought that low, low weight. For a client, this can be concerning and defeating—and understandably so. Every client gets scared when her body starts to gain a little bit of weight. Thankfully, she has me as her full-time coach to assure her that this, indeed, is normal.

Today, Julie weighs a very healthy 179 pounds. She works to maintain a five-to ten-pound "window" of grace. For someone this tall, a five- to ten-pound window is perfectly acceptable. For someone shorter—for example, under five feet, five inches tall—an acceptable window may be three to six pounds.

This slight rebound of weight should be expected and not ever seen as failure. Often my clients—and this may pertain to you as well—are diehard about getting to a low number. They work their food plan and overexert themselves with intense workouts. Remember, it's important that whatever you do to lose weight, you are willing to do long term. Whatever you start, are you willing to continue?

Julie's weight range is very acceptable. Remember, I had mentioned to you that my lowest weight was 142 pounds, but as I have pointed out, that was not a healthy number for me. That was merely a skinny number that I could not have maintained.

Now, my window range for my weight is between 168 and 178 pounds. My body is happy here. I am still lean looking. But most importantly, I am healthy, I am confident, I am self-assured, and I love myself. The workouts I did to compete in bodybuilding, I no longer do. To be blunt, I am living my life, working-out because it clears my head, and maintaining my weight without stress or anxiety.

THIS is where I want you to land as well. I want you to be joyful, not anxious about your weight, and to execute a food plan that fits into your NEW life. This is where contentment occurs. So do not fear if you hit an extremely low weight and then slightly rebound. You will NOT rebound to your starting weight, unless you choose to revert to your old life, old behaviors, and old choices. But a slight weight gain to a healthy, maintainable number should be expected. Remember, you're still winning, my dear friend. Also remember, success truly isn't about the number on the scale. True success is doing the internal work, conquering what led to your weight issue, and finding peace and love with how you treat your body.

Chapter 40

Something Doesn't Feel Right

I never know when body dysmorphia will hit, although I can now identify why it hits me. For me, baggy clothing will trigger this horrible feeling in my head. And suddenly, I feel like I am 250 pounds again!

I know you've heard the term before: body dysmorphia. But did you realize this disorder is classified as a mental illness? We'll cover why in a moment, but first, let's talk about this huge misconception that you will have during your weight-loss journey and, at times, into maintenance.

Sometimes you will feel it coming. Ladies, during your cycle, you will often feel down, blue, depressed, and apathetic about the work you have done. But even worse, you may look in the mirror or catch a glimpse of your reflection, and you will "see" the old you, the heavier you—the YOU that you have worked so hard to move away from. Other times, body dysmorphia will just hit you out of nowhere. Sadly, it will happen, and you may have a day or multiple days of truly NOT seeing your progress and you will become discouraged. Some even give up when body dysmorphia strikes.

Know this: body dysmorphia is temporary! It will go away. But if, after a few days or week, you still feel you are suffering, please talk to someone or even see your primary care physician. I have never had a client who has needed to go that extreme, but as I mentioned, body dysmorphia is classified as a mental illness, like depression and anxiety. Never, ever feel alone.

When body dysmorphia strikes, you will likely obsess over your flaws, focus only on the negative, and pick apart your body. You will spend an obsessive amount of time focusing on the 5 percent that you feel is "bad" about your body, rather than thinking rationally and recognizing the 95 percent that is fantastic. Your thoughts are disordered during this time.

If you choose to talk to a professional about your feelings or thoughts, you will likely be treated with a combination of medicines and behavioral therapy. The latter is vitally important, because behavioral therapy assists you in changing your thought process.

Most of my clients need some coaching to once again be able to recognize their efforts—both mentally and physically.

Here are a few quick tips and ideas that I use with my full-time clients:

1. When body dysmorphia hits, I ask the client if she is still wearing her "old" clothes. Has she taken the time to shop for new clothing that now fits her transitioning body? A lot of clients don't want to invest in new clothes until they hit their goal weight. I remind them that buying new clothes as they transform is a very important part of accepting the incredibly hard work they have done thus far. Being able to buy new clothes in a smaller size is a physical and mental reward. Knowing that you are down a size or two in clothing can motivate you to continue the path. It can be as simple as purchasing a few new bras, shirts, and pants. This doesn't have to be a wardrobe overhaul. The danger of NOT buying new clothes is twofold. First, you won't experience the joy of shopping for new, smaller clothes, but you also are "hiding" in your old clothing. No one will be able to see the massive transformation you have executed, and you will be staring back at the old you in the mirror, in your old clothes, daily. By doing this, your brain hasn't gotten accustomed to "see-

ing" you smaller. Your brain has some catching up to do; it needs to see and accept that you truly are smaller. You know in your heart that you are. But it takes time for your brain to play catch-up. Additionally, it's vitally important that you receive external affirmation. This won't happen if you are "hiding" and "swimming" in your old baggy clothing.

2. When a client complains of body dysmorphia, I quickly ask her if she was on plan the day or night prior. Sometimes, an unplanned treat meal or simply choosing to be off-plan will lead to negative body dysmorphia thoughts the next day. You may suddenly think you look fat when you were simply off-plan, and that action alone has you spinning.

There are several simple questions you need to ask yourself when you feel this way. Here are a few:

1. Why do I feel ugly today? or Why do I feel big today?

2. Why do I feel stuck today?

3. Why am I spending an obsessive amount of time focusing on the negative?

4. What positive thoughts or "wins" about my journey should I be focusing on, rather than the negative?

5. Am I able to realize this false reality will pass?

The last point is likely the most important. If you cannot recognize that your current perception of your body is false, and that these thoughts will pass, then please seek medical assistance either with a primary care physician or a licensed therapist. Your thoughts and mindset about your journey will absolutely affect your progress, so do not be afraid to admit you need more help.

Chapter 41

Uncovering Your NEW YOU

It's very possible that sometime under the age of six, you experienced a traumatic event that shaped who you are and what you believe. You may be vividly aware of this moment, or like me, you don't remember a defining moment quite that young.

However, as I have mentioned, I remember being called "Big Bertha" at the age of nine!

THAT was my first defining moment, and it certainly was not the last, that shaped who I truly believed I was. I absorbed the title of "Big Bertha" deep in my brain, and I manifested what I believed a "Big Bertha" looked like, for decades. To add insult to injury, I was super tall, wasn't comfortable in my skin, didn't look like the tiny cheerleaders at school, and never had a boyfriend as all the skinny girls did, so I assumed I was fat. All these thoughts deep in my brain were solidified before I even went to college.

While attending the University of Cincinnati, the rollercoaster diet ride continued. I would gain and then lose a lot of weight. At my heaviest weight in college, and clearly not my happiest of years, I knew my college roommate and others were calling me names behind my back and saying hurtful words that I believed were truths about me, so I continued to manifest "Big Bertha"!

After losing quite a bit of weight, a male college friend of mine complimented me by saying, "Wow, you no longer have tree trunks for legs!" It was quite the back-handed compliment that honestly didn't help or flatter me.

Adding insult to injury, I saw my grandmother who was living in Cincinnati while I was finishing up at the University of Cincinnati. I remember exactly where I was standing in my Aunt Kay's house, and exactly what I was wearing—light-colored jeans that I was so thrilled to be wearing because I had lost weight.

My grandmother was in the dining room. I had entered the living room, and she took one look at me and said, "It's such a shame that you inherited the Jewett [her last name] big legs!"

Once again, even in a lower weight, I was continuing to manifest the "Big Bertha" label from when I was nine years old.

I never felt good enough or pretty enough! And it was constantly wrecking me inside!

From my twenties to thirties, I worked so hard to "hide" Big Bertha. I hid her in amazing clothes and lots of girdles and tights. But as you can imagine, from what I've explained about my first marriage, that too had me believing I was still Big Bertha.

I had manifested Big Bertha. I was Big Bertha. All my negative thoughts, a lack of true love and acceptance, a lack of perceived attention I thought I needed from the opposite sex, the horrible words said by my first husband, and his perception of what his wife should have looked like, all made Big Bertha my reality.

Then, in my mid-thirties, I lost it all—accordingly to worldly standards. To be very clear, I fully believe this is when the Lord was trying to shake me, draw me closer to Him, and in turn allow me to hear the Holy Spirit.

I was a vice president at a local television station, owned by the New York Times, making incredible money. The New York Times sold all nine of their stations, and new station ownership came in and slowly replaced all VPs and department heads. I was one of the last to receive a severance package. I had minutes to pack up my office of seven years and head out the door.

My first marriage was failing. For over a year, I had worked the slow process of trying to encourage my first husband to engage with me to renew our marriage. We did months of couple's therapy, but nothing was working. I felt trapped and scared. No one in my family had ever been divorced, and I knew my father wouldn't agree. Even worse, I feared I would be disowned.

I felt stuck between two different lives—both in my marriage and certainly internally. I knew my marriage would never be what it could, and I constantly felt stuck in an overweight body. I wanted out of both my marriage and my body!

I was desperate to get out of my life with my first husband, but I didn't have a clear path. He wasn't accepting that I was dead serious on a divorce. Twice in this time period, I contemplated suicide. The first attempt I considered was a bottle of sleeping pills. The other near attempt was in my car. I was driving over a very high and long bridge and had multiple thoughts of driving so fast that my car would go over the bridge barrier and hit the water, and I would most likely die. Thankfully, I never fully executed either attempt. I knew it was up to me to raise my three children, and I couldn't leave them.

Finally, my first husband left the family house. Our marriage was over. He needed to find his own way, find his own job, and provide for himself.

A few months later, my father gave his permission for me to divorce. Four days later, my father died horrifically. For two decades, he had dealt with water at the base of the brain. A stent had been inserted, but as quickly as fluids would drain from his body, it would produce more. This caused an imbalance that led to him falling quite often, and he would fall hard due to having only one arm. Add on the fact that he was six foot eight, and he would fall far. It was gut-wrenching to watch this powerful man, known and respected all through his community, come undone. The last fall he had was in my parents' house in Camp Hill, Pennsylvania. He fell backward down two steps onto the wood floors of the family room.

Unconscious, he was rushed to the hospital, his head was shaved, and surgeons drained the mass of blood collecting in his brain. The doctors then broke the news to my mother. Even if he did wake up, the mass of blood was so incredibly large that it had pushed the right side of his brain into his left, and it would never return to its rightful side. He likely wouldn't ever feed himself, he perhaps would not walk again, and the worst part was he likely wouldn't remember who we were. Ultimately, we had to make the decision to take my father off life support.

So, in nine short months, I lost it all. I lost my marriage, my wildly successful career, and my father.

But this is when the most incredible journey began. I was back to ground zero. I was being forced to rebuild. I had no choice other than to deal with the iceberg that I had made for myself. I finally had the opportunity to be free from one of my "dead" lives (my marriage), and I had all the power to start dealing with my decades-long weight issue.

The summer my father died; I did a lot of self-reflection; growth always comes from this. While I thought I had lost everything, I realized I had only lost money, a dead marriage, and an ailing father. I rested in faith, knowing would I spend eternity with my father, so very honestly, that was oddly easy to process. Losing my job crushed my ego, but through self-reflection, I realized nothing truly good ever comes from our egos. And as for losing my first marriage, I knew I had an opportunity to rebuild from the ashes.

Losing everything presented me with an opportunity to rebuild victoriously and finally heal. Now, it's important to note that my weight at this time was not a large issue; I was on the lower end of the weight rollercoaster, and it would be several more years of destructive eating and drinking that would lead me to my highest weight. But I firmly believe God was lining things up systematically for me to conquer so that ultimately my mess (weight issue) could be my message and therefore help thousands of others.

When I began writing this book, it forced me to walk through a process of remembering and rediscovering why I chose certain behaviors and why I chose food and alcohol. Through that discovery process, I finally was able to see how I had truly manifested Big Bertha. I alone had given life to Big Bertha. However, the people around me, the people I was supposed to be trusting, "watered" the seed of Big Bertha and inadvertently gave life to the false perception. This was continually occurring from the ages of nine to thirty-five.

You are staring at likely one of the largest opportunities of your life—losing the weight and uncovering the most authentic, vibrant, and beYOUtiful version of you. You've been waiting and wishing and hoping for this moment, and the Lord has been waiting for you to do the work, one step at a time. The Lord has orchestrated a season of preparation for you, just as He did for me. Perhaps buying this book was the start of the season of preparation, or perhaps the book is the last piece of the puzzle for you. But no one will do the work for you, no one is coming to save you, and no one is coming to execute this for you.

Likely the hardest part of your journey will be getting below the surface of your weight issue. There's no ignoring the iceberg and what lies beneath the water. If you choose to ignore it and what truly caused and fed into your weight issue, you will continue the weight-loss rollercoaster; you will never heal your relationship with food. If you want true victory, as you walk your journey, you must deal with the emotions, the excuses, and the food or alcohol abuse, and really define what led to all of this. Even more important, you must establish ways of successfully coping and navigating your new life without emotionally eating or drinking (replacement behaviors). Your reliance on food or alcohol will never fully be cured; it simply goes into remission, with you being more educated and more powerful than the old habit.

Your paramount goal is to heal your relationship with food. There is no room for healing until you uncover the reasons why you turn to food or alcohol. You can't heal half-way. You must dig deep and be honest about the iceberg. Let me clear, healing is not a "one and done" process. It's not a decade-long process. It's a daily process for the rest of your life. This isn't a forgive-and-forget situation. You can't just walk away from food as you would a friend who has abused your relationship. Food and alcohol are always lurking. You simply cannot live without food. Frankly, food is your friend. So, it's YOUR responsibility to establish NEW healthy boundaries.

A great starting point is to go back and reread the chapters about the iceberg. Each time you read those words, you will uncover more and more of your thoughts, emotions, and memories—the good, the bad, and the really ugly! Each time you reread the chapters, you will go to a deeper level of the iceberg. This is vitally important for your growth. If you enjoy journaling, write down your thoughts every time you read those chapters. Or you can work through them with a licensed therapist. I cannot stress this enough: there is NO avoiding this part of the journey. You cannot avoid it if you want to truly heal your relationship with food and never diet again.

Also remember, it's vitally important throughout your journey that you fail. I know that sounds counterproductive, but it's the complete truth. Each time you fail and revert fully or partially to old habits, you must see it as an opportunity for growth. I'm nearly a decade into my journey, and I still fail. And honestly, when I fail, I am able to laugh about it now. I have moments, days, or multiple days when I lose my footing. But every single time, I will sit quietly and review why I believe I failed and how to establish new ways, new coping skills, to not repeat that failure. Each time you allow yourself to fail, go back and reread the chapters on navigating the grey and recovering after you do indeed fall.

The longer you persevere in this journey, the more your goodness, your true purpose, and your beYOUtiful self will be revealed. There will be painful days, weeks, and months. Remember, the message is always the same: Once you hit rock bottom, there's nowhere to go but up. But you must choose UP because you are destined for something better, something glorious, powerful, and amazing. Remember, you aren't duct taped to the "chair" of life!

This is also a season when your life-long perceptions of who you were will fall to the wayside. Trust me here. You may not realize it or feel it, but it's happening.

Believe this: You have a divine mission, but none of that will occur if your don't do all the preparation now and walk the journey.

I've said this many, many times: I feel as if my life has been a series of wrong decisions, doing things backwards and full of mistakes. Many of these choices and wrong decisions led me to a "Big Bertha" life. Now, while I feel that I've done everything backwards, I have no regrets for my hasty decisions, wrong decisions, years of paving the wrong path, and years of rollercoaster dieting. Each one of these messes has led to something amazing.

I've had people ask me if I regret my first marriage. When they ask this, I first think about or visualize my three children. My answer is, always and adamantly, NO. I have three fantastic, incredible, world-changing children from that mess. I am incredibly proud of the men and woman they have become. I am honored by their determination and dedication and the paths they have chosen.

Others ask me if I regret all the diet pills and the money I spent on plastic surgery. My answer is always the same: NO. That mess has made me a much better coach. It's made me relatable.

Then there are some who ask, do I miss working in television? That answer is mixed. Yes and no. I liked the fast pace of television. I liked the people and the high-performing energy. In some ways, news is like working in an emergency room. You never know what you're going to face each day, yet everyone comes to together to meet incredibly tight deadlines and produce something amazing. However, if I hadn't left local television, my ego would now be through the roof. I likely would have never met Stephen and never realized my divine purpose, the beYOUtiful path I was meant to pave.

Your exciting season of preparation has already begun. Believe it. Receive it. It's time to create the NEW, beYOUtiful YOU! You are about to cross over to a new life, so let's address that next.

Chapter 42

Killing the Old

Big Bertha officially died October 17, 2020, while writing this book. I literally said out loud: "Big Bertha is dead." I am not Big Bertha; I never was. For forty years, I had allowed other people's words to feed into a stupid nine-year-old boy's comment, and unknowingly and for far too long, I had chosen to manifest a false reality OF ME. Sadly, it had shaped decades of my life.

After exactly forty years, Big Bertha died. She suddenly had no role or strength over my life and never would again.

Now it's time for you to recognize your new life, your new you, and to fully kill the old. So here we go!

A word of warning: this may not be easy. This process within your journey to beYOUtiful may take a while. It may be painful and yet at times hilarious. Do not feel that you must complete this task in a day, let alone a month or year. Lots of self-reflection will be required, and you will have to dig deep. But trust me, it is completely worth it.

Think deeply about these things:

> What words, comments, slights, and insults are you allowing to manifest and rule your life, your destiny?

What do you think occurred at a young age that led to your weight issue?

Was there a defining moment later in life that shaped your life and weight gain?

How do you deal with the continual negative thoughts you have? Do you believe those negative thoughts?

If you and I were on a phone call right now and I asked you to describe your own beliefs and thoughts about yourself, what would you tell me?

Do you realize that if you have suffered from other's people's words, back-handed comments, negative attention, or even lack of attention, you have likely created a false identity for yourself?

Have you allowed others to feed into this defining moment? This could be a sibling, a stranger, parent(s), a husband, or even a close friend.

Now, most importantly, do you realize you have all the control and capacity to change your false identity and usher in truth? You really, truly do have all the power.

Step 1: Acceptance. Accept that people and kids are mean. The words that come out of their mouths can be brutal, cutting, and frankly, life-altering—accept this. If you feel your parents contributed to where you are now, accept that, hopefully, they were doing their best. They only had the capacity to provide for you emotionally, based on their own life experiences. You can't change what has happened to you or been said to you. Accept it and focus on Step 2.

Step 2: Awareness. Be aware that you have misinterpreted your manifestation. This was a small mistake on your part that you've allowed to grow uncontrollably. Remember, it's a small mistake. SMALL. Can you own up to the fact you likely manifested a false identity for yourself?

My brother-in-law, John, recently shared a family picture of me, ironically, from the fourth grade—that fateful grade when I was called "Big Bertha"!

I showed it to my husband, Stephen, and we laughed. I was so skinny. My tummy was flat, and my face wasn't full. But I was tall. Brian's "Big Bertha" comment, I now believe, was because I was just shy of five feet tall in the fourth grade. I was taller than every boy in my class for a very long time. But for forty years I haven't been able to accept that very likely his comment was about my height. I had misinterpreted his comment and manifested it incorrectly. For forty years, I carried around a false perception of myself.

Step 3: Adjustment. Now work to kill your false perception! It must die 100 percent. This is the hardest step. It will not happen overnight. You must plant a seed into your brain and let it grow on your own terms, and this will take time. However, I hope and pray it won't take you forty years, as it did for me. This is also the step where you may want to seriously consider professional counseling.

Let me help you fast-track this step right now.

I want you to realize that even when we are presented with facts, they often don't change our minds. I am here to tell you that you are not the lies you currently believe about yourself. Yet your intelligent self may not see this clearly because others' thoughts and comments and your own negative thoughts have persuaded you to believe otherwise. Read that last sentence again.

Your brain is literally built to have a greater sensitivity to negative experiences and thoughts, I suppose, to allow us to recognize and keep us away from danger. However, that sets us all up for a bit of failure—consistent, overwhelming, daily negative self-talk. Shockingly, there is a five-to-one ratio of bad to good thoughts in our brain!

When you have recurring negative thought patterns, you cannot perform at a high or even NORMAL capacity. You are literally obsessed or trapped by negative thoughts. Your brain has a deep tendency to focus, replay, and remember only the negative thoughts or experiences you have. Sadly, your brain is wired to scout out the negativity. Even more concerning, your negative thoughts have energy and can literally rewire not only your brain, but also your cells and genes. Healing your relationship with food will never occur if you choose to focus on the abundance of negativity. And yes, friend, it's a choice to focus on the negative!

Every day we have about 12,000 to 60,000 thoughts. Now buckle up! Of those thoughts, 80 percent of them are negative and 95 percent of them are repeat thoughts. Our thoughts are literally on replay daily.

The false perception you have created for yourself (and others in your life have likely "watered") stems from negative thoughts. To kill your long-standing false perception of yourself, you must take actionable steps to counteract these negative thoughts. This exercise is vitally important to rewiring your brain to continually focus on the positive. No, the negative thoughts won't fully disappear, but you can choose to focus daily on the positive versus the negative.

You clearly know that positive thoughts make you feel happy, joyful, and optimistic. When these thoughts prevail, your cortisol decreases and the brain replaces serotonin. So conversely, imagine what all those negative thoughts are doing to your brain and body. It's literally making you sick— emotionally and physically.

The largest part of growth right now will come from hearing the negative thoughts in your head and then immediately stating the truth. It takes a conscious effort to do this, because for years or decades you have easily accepted the negative lie. It's easier to accept the negative lie because your brain is wired to scout out the negative! Now as soon as that negative thought comes into your head, be willing and open to immediately saying the truth.

As a coach to thousands, here are the lies I hear the most often:

1. **Negative thought:** I will be fat the rest of my life.
   Truth: No, my current state is a choice, and it's also a choice to choose a healthier lifestyle.

2. **Negative thought:** I'll never be able to kick alcohol and/or sugar out of my life.
   Truth: No, I have full control over my choices. I may need help

seeking out replacement behaviors or making better choices, but I have control over what I put in my mouth.

3. **Negative thought:** My mom/dad/spouse tells me I'm fat.
   Truth: This person is very likely projecting his or her own insecurities with weight or something else (I may not know exactly what) on me. The problem being projected on me (that I'm fat) is how this person tries to feel better. This comment is not about me, but rather the other person's insecurity.

Once you can consistently attack your negative thoughts, you need to realize that ultimately every one of us has a deeply ingrained desire to belong, in some way, to a larger "tribe." Additionally, we want to be just like everyone else.

All of my memories of being super tall led to my feeling alone. In middle school and high school, never being cast as the lead in a musical because I was so much taller than the male lead, not because of my vocal abilities, led to my feeling that I wasn't pretty enough to be the star. The mere fact that I was so tall meant that I always wore a larger size of clothing that all my friends. What a mess!

We are meant to bond with others, to earn respect, and to have the approval of our peers or parents. This is essential to our survival. So when we are cast out—when we are perhaps called a horrible name—we are separated emotionally from our "tribe," and we begin to manifest our false reality. This casting out can be minor, yet our brains don't know how to process that small comment, or it can be as vivid as abuse or rape.

You have allowed yourself to be condemned by others, according to your beliefs from a very young age of who you should be.

We don't always believe things because they are correct. We believe things that make us look good to the people around us or the people we deeply care about. So if you aren't being positively reinforced as a young child by peers or parents, you suddenly feel emotionally detached from your tribe. You feel different from your tribe, and in feeling different, you are feeling wrong. You don't fit in.

You feel isolated and wrong because you think you're too big, tall, short, fat, ugly, or stupid compared to those around you.

I've told you my sisters are ten and seven years older than I am. I grew up admiring them, their beauty, and their clothes. I also remember the size of clothing they wore, which for many of my childhood years was much smaller than mine. I just wanted to be like them. But at a young age (I believe age twelve), I was wearing a larger size than they were. My bone and muscular structure was larger than theirs and obviously, still to this day, I am taller and larger (not in a bad way) than they are. Growing up, my idea was that I was flawed because I didn't look like them; I wasn't built like they were, so I was bad. I didn't fit the Kerr mold. So, in my young brain, I was the token fat Kerr daughter.

Talk about debilitating. Talk about impressionable, and talk about feeling different from your tribe. This never was my sisters' fault, and honestly, they probably never knew I felt this way. I don't blame them at all. It is what it is. But these internal thoughts certainly piled onto that horrible "Big Bertha" comment. Not only was I separated from my tribe at school, but that also carried out into my home life for decades!

When you feel different or separated from your tribe, a crack occurs inside you. In this crack is where your seed of false reality has planted in your brain, and soon you're manifesting a very false perception of yourself.

NOTE: For many of us this does occur in childhood; however, I've seen this happen to adult clients as well after some traumatic event, such as rape or a nasty divorce!

How do think you were separated from your tribe as a child? And how do you feel separated from your tribe now? What do you always say about yourself now? What do you say about your appearance? Do you still feel separated from your tribe, right now, as an adult?

You must change your own perception of yourself, and like I said, this is time-consuming but completely worth it. By doing this, you aren't denying your thoughts, your feelings, or your brain's reality, but you are going to change the lenses you have chosen to remember these thoughts, feelings, and emotions.

Think about it this way. You have glued all these thoughts and false realities to yourself like superglue. Now, you must slowly pick the glue off. I know it sounds painful, but very honestly, it's going to feel amazing to see yourself completely differently. You are literally freeing yourself and your thoughts, and then you can usher in and fully accept your new beYOUtiful you.

How?

We are going to flip the script. We first attacked the negative thoughts; now let's attack the false perceptions!

My false perception:

I am so tall that no man will like me. All the tall men choose short women. Men must be attracted only to short women.

Flip the script:

I am so tall that short women wish they had my long legs and height. Tall men love tall women. It makes a man feel strong and powerful to be standing next to a tall woman.

My false perception:

I am unlovable at a size 12, 14, or 22.

Flip the script:

A real man will love a woman at any size. It's not the number on the scale that matters. Her confidence, joy, and happiness are paramount, and they are what make her attractive.

I want you to start listing out your negative, false perceptions, and then I want you to write out the positive reality. I want you to flip the negative perception in your head. This is the only way to begin freeing yourself, your thoughts, and your long-term false perceptions of yourself. This exercise will manifest your thoughts and actions so you will see yourself as you never have before.

Wow!! This is exciting!

You will finally be free.

And even more exciting is that you will grow into a beYOUtiful version of you—the authentic, free, and purposeful YOU.

PS: R.I.P Big Bertha. I hope you don't rest in peace.

PPS: If you have children, I hope and pray you are raising them to be super-inclusive of the tribe around them. No one deserves to be haunted by two words or a negative label for forty years.

Chapter 43

Being BeYOUtiful

Your weight loss is the byproduct of doing all the mental and emotional work outlined in these chapters. The easy part is following the food plan. The true transformation isn't about losing weight. It's being aware of how you got here, dealing with the past, forgiving yourself and others, and then boldly uncovering the most beYOUtiful version of you. And what you see now, on the outside, is merely the reward of all your hard, internal work!

Even more exciting is that you and I stand in agreement that healing our relationship with food is a daily process!

I hope and pray that your beYOUtiful life will be wildly different from the life of false perceptions that you have been living for years. Listen to me, friend—your life can be wildly different if you just choose to never stop, never stop healing, and always remember to put yourself first!

I am so excited and convinced that your life will be radically changed that I want to hear about it. Please find my contact information in the appendix and send me an email!

I am super proud of you!

I want you to fully realize that while you've done a massive amount of work and have likely grown and developed into a new person, the journey will never be done. There isn't a finish line. A wellness journey is never "one and done." You are a living being; you are full of energy. Let's simplify this: You have houseplants. What happens if you don't water them? They die, obviously. You are just like a houseplant. You must continually "water" yourself, work on your emotions, quiet the negative script in your head, and work to maintain your emotional strength, mindset, and now your lower weight. Remember, if you aren't growing, you're dying. It's that simple.

Keep growing. Keep fighting any pulls back to your old life, your old behavioral choices, and any reminders of the old perceptions you had about your body and your life.

ALWAYS remember that you are a child of God. From the day you were born, He has been fighting for you. While it may have seemed through your hard years that He was quiet, silent, and nowhere near, He has never left you, and He truly wants you to beYOUtiful.

Now, we aren't done. You need resources, recipes, meal plans, goal-setting guidance, and much more. So enjoy the next section, and remember that you can reach out to me at any time; my contact information is included as well.

Welcome to the start of your new life—it's BeYOUtiful!

Section 4

Appendix

Appendix
Table of Contents

Contact Martha:

Email: martha@beyoutifulthebook.com

Website: bemarthafit.com

Martha's Recipe Website:

recipes.bemarthafit.com

Lean Protein Examples

Lean skinless chicken breast or turkey breast

Lean pork loin

Flank Steak

96% lean ground turkey

96% lean ground beef

White fish

Shrimp

Complex Carb Examples

Quinoa

Brown Rice

Couscous

Sweet Potato

Black Beans

Healthy Fat Examples

Avocado

Plain nuts

Nut butters

Hummus

Steady-State 1,500-Calorie Plan

Average Calories: 1,500 | Protein: 175 | Fat: 26 | Carbs: 176

Breakfast Options: Pick one and alternate:

1. ¾ cup of oats and 2x the water, microwaved. Add in 1 scoop of whey protein. Top with either: ½ cup of berries or cherries or ½ banana

2. Kodiak Cakes: ½ cup of Kodiak Protein Packed Mix. Mix with ½ cup of mix and ½ cup of water, 2 full eggs. May use: sugar free syrup, spray butter and either ½ cup of berries or ½ cup of bananas. May only have 2x a week.

3. 2x week: 1 egg, 4 egg whites and 1 cup veggies. PLUS: one slice Dave's Killer Bread (thin sliced). Small amount of sugar free jelly and spray butter.

Morning Snack Options: Pick one and alternate:

1. 2 low-fat cheese sticks with 1/2 cup of grapes and 1 protein shake.

2. Lemon Muffins, recipe provided. Eat 3

3. 2 flavored rice cakes and 1 cup low-fat cottage cheese.

Lunch Guidelines:

4 ounces lean protein, 1 cup of veggies and ½ cup complex carb.

Please see guideline sheet below for list of approved options

Afternoon Snack Options: Pick one and alternate:

1. Approved protein bar (see guideline sheet)

2. Coffee drink: 1 premade protein shake and 1 cup of cold brew (no more than 5 calories). Also, 1.5 Tbsp of natural peanut butter.

Dinner Guidelines:

4 ounces lean protein and 2 cups of veggies.

Please see guideline sheet below for list of approved options

Evening Snack Option:

1. Halo Top Ice Cream: 2 servings
2. Protein shake
3. Make your own protein ice cream: 1.5 scoops whey protein, ½-¾ cup unsweetened almond milk. Freeze for 45 minutes. May add a small amount of sugar-free whipped topping.

APPROVED LEAN PROTEINS

Chicken breast
Lean ground turkey
Lean ground beef
Flank steak 2x a week
Salmon 2x a week
Shrimp
White fish
Pork Loin

APPROVED PROTEIN BARS

BSN Crisp
Quest
No Cow
Grenade
Combat
Kirkland
Oh Yeah One
Pure Protein
Think Thin High Protein
Fit Factor

APPROVED WHEY PROTEIN

Quest
ISO 100
Pure Protein
Designer Whey
PE Science
Garden of Life
Bownar
Paleo Protein
About Time
Optimum Nutrition Gold Standard
Evolve
Olympian Labs Pea Protein
Health Warriors Superfood

APPROVED COMPLEX CARBS

Brown rice
Sweet potatoes
Couscous
Quinoa

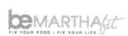

Steady-State 1,800-Calorie Plan

Average Calories: 1,800 | Protein: 190 | Fat: 52 | Carbs: 260

Breakfast Options: Pick one and alternate:

1. ⅔ cup of oats and 2x the water, microwaved. Add in 1 scoop of whey protein. Top with either: ½ cup of berries or cherries or ½ banana

2. Cottage Cheese Pancakes, recipe provided. Recipe makes one serving!

3. 3 full eggs, make any style. May add in veggies and SMALL amount of low fat cheese. PLUS: one slice Dave's Killer Bread or Ezekiel Bread.

Morning Snack Options: Pick one and alternate:

1. 1 Oikos Triple Zero Greek yogurt (black label), medium apple and 15 plain almonds.

2. Pumpkin Muffins, recipe provided. Eat 3

Lunch Guidelines:

5.5 ounces lean protein, 1 cup of veggies and ½ cup complex carb. Please see guideline sheet below for list of approved options

Afternoon Snack Options: Pick one and alternate:

1. Approved protein bar (see guideline sheet). Also, 1 TBSP natural peanut butter.

2. Chocolate Kodiak Protein Muffins, recipe provided. Eat 3 with small apple.

Dinner Guidelines:

5.5 ounces lean protein, 1 cup of veggies and ¾ cup complex carb. Please see guideline sheet below for list of approved options

Evening Snack Option:

1. Halo Top Ice Cream: 1 serving
2. Protein shake

APPROVED LEAN PROTEINS

Chicken breast
Lean ground turkey
Lean ground beef
Flank steak 2x a week
Salmon 2x a week
Shrimp
White fish
Pork Loin

APPROVED PROTEIN BARS

BSN Crisp
Quest
No Cow
Grenade
Combat
Kirkland
Oh Yeah One
Pure Protein
Think Thin High Protein
Fit Factor

APPROVED WHEY PROTEIN

Quest
ISO 100
Pure Protein
Designer Whey
PE Science
Garden of Life
Bownar
Paleo Protein
About Time
Optimum Nutrition Gold Standard
Olympian Labs Pea Protein
Health Warriors Superfood

APPROVED COMPLEX CARBS

Sweet potatoes
Couscous
Quinoa

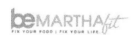

Steady-State 2,100-Calorie Plan

Average Calories: 2,100 | Protein: 190 | Fat: 52 | Carbs: 260

Breakfast Options: Pick one and alternate:

1. ¾ cup of oats and 2x the water, microwaved. Add in 1 scoop of whey protein. Top with either: ½ cup of berries or cherries or ½ banana

2. Kodiak Cakes: Combine: ½ cup of Kodiak Protein Packed Mix, ½ cup of water and 2 full eggs. May use: sugar free syrup, spray butter and either ½ cup of berries or ½ cup of bananas. May only have 2x a week.

3. Cottage Cheese Pancakes, recipe provided. Recipe makes one serving!

4. 1 cup Kashi Go cereal, unsweetened almond milk and 2 eggs, any style OR 1 protein shake. Only 2x week.

5. 4 full eggs, make any style. May add in veggies and SMALL amount of low fat cheese. PLUS: one slice Dave's Killer Bread or Ezekiel Bread.

Morning Snack Options: Pick one and alternate:

1. 2 low-fat cheese sticks with 1 cup of grapes and 1 protein shake.

2. Blueberry Muffins, recipe provided. Eat 3.

3. 2 flavored rice cakes and 1 cup lowfat cottage cheese.

Lunch Guidelines:

5.5 ounces lean protein, 1 cup of veggies and 1 cup complex carb. Please see guideline sheet below for list of approved options

Afternoon Snack Options: Pick one and alternate:

1. Approved protein bar (see guideline sheet). Also, medium apple and 1.5 TBS natural peanut butter.

2. Coffee drink: 1 premade protein shake and 1 cup of cold brew (no more than 5 calories). Also, 2 TBS of natural peanut butter and 1 cheese stick

Dinner Guidelines:

5 ounces lean protein, 1 cup of veggies and 1 cup complex carb. Please see guideline sheet below for list of approved options

Evening Snack Option:

1. Halo Top Ice Cream: 2 servings
2. Protein shake
3. 1 cup low fat cottage cheese.

APPROVED LEAN PROTEINS

Chicken breast
Lean ground turkey
Lean ground beef
Flank steak 2x a week
Salmon 2x a week
Shrimp
White fish
Pork Loin

APPROVED PROTEIN BARS

BSN Crisp
Quest
No Cow
Grenade
Combat
Kirkland
Oh Yeah One
Pure Protein
Think Thin High Protein
Fit Factor

APPROVED WHEY PROTEIN

Quest
ISO 100
Pure Protein
Designer Whey
PE Science
Garden of Life
Bownar
Paleo Protein
About Time
Evolve
Olympian Labs Pea Protein
Health Warriors Superfood

APPROVED COMPLEX CARBS

Brown rice
Sweet potatoes
Couscous
Quinoa

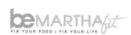

Healthy Eating Blueprint

BREAKFAST - **Protein and Complex Carb**
        300 calories | 35g carbs| 20g protein | 10g fats

AM SNACK - **Protein and Complex Carb**
        200-300 calories | 12g carbs|
        20g protein | 5g fats

LUNCH - **Protein and Complex Carb or Protein and Healthy Fats**
        300 calories | 35g carbs|
        25g protein | 5g fats

PM SNACK - **Protein and "Pick Me Up"**
        200 calories | 20g carbs |
        25g protein | 5g fats

DINNER - **Protein and Veggies**
        250 - 300 calories | 35g carbs|
        20g protein | 10g fats

Note: To accurately track calories and macros (macros are carbs, fats, and proteins), you will want to download a free app such as My Fitness Pal and get a food scale. When meal prepping, be sure to weigh your food on the food scale so you can accurately log meals into the app. The app will show you a breakdown of your macros and help you track your goals.

Yes/No/Maybe Food List

The Yes Foods

Meat and Fish

beef
buffalo
chicken
clams
duck
eggs
game meats
salmon
goat
halibut
lamb

lobster
mahi-mahi
mussels
pork loin
red snapper
scallops
swordfish
turkey—white meat
tuna
veal

Vegetables

artichoke
asparagus
broccoli
brussels sprouts
cabbage
carrots--minimal
cauliflower
celery
collards
cucumber
eggplant
garlic, ginger

green beans
kale
leeks
mushrooms
onions
parsnips
peppers
radishes
snow peas—minimal
spinach
tomato—minimal
turnips

Dairy

half and half
heavy cream
cheese—usually low-fat

cottage cheese
non-fat plain Greek yogurt

Nuts/Seeds/Butter

almond butter
coconut butter
100% cacao
macadamias
hazelnuts
flax
chia

hemp
pecans
pistachios
walnuts
sesame seeds
tahani

Fats/Oils

butter-sparingly
spray butter
ghee
avocado

coconut oil/milk
flax oil
olive oil
sesame oil

Beverages

water
mineral water seltzer
club soda
coffee
espresso

unsweet tea (green, black, herbal)
unsweetened almond, cashew, or coconut milk
coffee

The No Foods

Vegetables

corn, white
potatoes
winter squash

Fruits

See the "sometimes" list

Refined/Simple Carbs

bread
bagels
breadsticks
brownies
cake
candy
cereal/granola
chips

cookies
crackers
croissants
cupcakes
muffins
pasta
pastries
pizza

Beverages

alcohol
sugary coffee drinks

milks
soda

Sauces

any sauce with sugar in it
soy sauce (you can use coconut aminos)

Limit Foods

Vegetables

try to limit the following to 1 cup a day: beets, butternut squash, pumpkin

Fruits

any berries: blueberry, strawberry, blackberry
apples—ideally green

Grains/Legumes

black beans
chickpeas

quinoa
red beans

Sauces and Condiments

- Coconut Secrets Amino Acids
- Coconut Secrets Garlic Sauce
- Ginger People Ginger Peanut Sauce
- Trader Joe's Green Dragon
- G. Hughes Marinades
- G. Hughes Sugar Free bbq Sauce
- Maple Grove Farms Sugar Free Maple Syrup
- Kraft Avocado Oil Mayo
- Blue Palate Low Sodium Spaghetti Sauce
- Opa Dressings
- Bolthouse Dressings
- Walden Farms Dressings and Syrups
- Simply 60 Dressings
- Panera Poppy Seed Dressing
- Green Mountain Gringo Salsa
- Taco Bell Mild Sauce
- Wuju Hot Sauce
- Sriracha Hot Sauce
- Dave's Gourmet Hot Sauces
- Mustard
- Sugar-Free Ketchup
- Smucker's Sugar-Free Preserves

Note: Sauces and condiments should be low-calorie, low-sodium, and sugar-free.

Spices and Seasonings

- Mrs. Dash
- Oh My Spices
- Flavor God
- McCormick's Perfect Pinch Salt Free Seasonings
- Flavor Mate Salt Free Seasonings
- NoSalt Original Sodium-Free Salt Alternative (use sparingly)
- Pink Himalayan salt

Note: All salt-free, sugar-free spices are approved. (All single ingredient spices such as onion powder, garlic powder, basil, oregano, crushed red pepper flakes, etc., are approved.)

High-Fat 1,400-Calorie Plan

Average Calories: 1,420 | Protein: 152 | Fat: 70 | Carbs: 65

Breakfast Options: Pick one and alternate:

1. Quick Crunch "Cereal"; recipe provided. Eat 1 serving.
2. 3 full egg with 3 pieces of nitrate free turkey bacon and 1 cup of spinach/greens. May make into an omelet.
3. Apple Sage Turkey Breakfast Sausage, recipe provided. Eat 3 patties
4. Low carb waffle/pancake: combine 2 eggs, 1 scoop protein and ¼ tsp. baking powder and any spices you would like. Changing protein powders gives lots of variety. Blend and make into a waffle or pancakes. May also top with spray butter or sugar free syrup or heavy whipped topping and ½ cup of berries. These toast well so you can make a big batch and throw in the toaster the morning of.

Morning Snack Options: Pick one and alternate:

1. Low Carb Double Chocolate Muffins, recipe provided. Eat 1
2. Protein shake and .5 ounces of almonds (about 10 almonds)
3. Approved protein bar and 1 small apple. Please see guideline sheet below for approved options

Lunch Guidelines:

5 ounces protein and 1 cup of veggies. Note: You do not have to use lean meat only. You can use salmon and steak here. No corn, sweet peas or carrots. Please see guideline sheet below for list of approved options

You may make this a salad. Use 2 cups of spinach and filler veggies with your protein. Use Bolthouse or Walden Farms dressing. Pay attention to serving size on label of dressing

Afternoon Snack Options: Pick one and alternate:

1. Bedtime Nut Butter Pudding, recipe provided. Top with 1 ounce of walnuts
2. 2 Plant power thins with 4 TBSP of hummus
3. Guacamole: Use raw veggies such as peppers, cucumber and celery as "chips" Eat 1 serving which is ½ o f recipe provided.
4. One low carb mission wrap (about 110 cals.) Plus 4 oz low sodium boars head turkey deli meat with greens. Can add 1 TBSP Olive Oil Mayo or Bolthouse dressing.

Dinner Guidelines:

5 ounces protein and 1 cup of veggies. No corn, sweet peas or carrots. Please see guideline sheet below for list of approved options

Evening Snack Option:

1. Halo Top Ice Cream: 1.5 servings
2. Protein shake
3. Chef Casey's Cake in Mug, recipe provided.

Plantpower Bread Thins. YOU CAN ALSO GET THESE AT WEGMAN'S! https://www.outeraislegourmet.com/?gclid=EAIaIQobChMI8tX0yNCl4wIVz-FYNCh08EQSxEAAYASAAEgISbvD_BwE

Instant Keto Cereal: https://www.amazon.com/gp/product/B07JP79VQZ/ref=ppx_yo_dt_b_asin_title_o08_s00?ie=UTF8&psc=1

APPROVED LEAN PROTEINS	APPROVED PROTEIN BARS
Chicken breast	Atkins Snack Bar
Lean ground turkey	Quest Hero Bars
Lean ground beef	No Cow
Flank steak	Quest Beyond Cereal Bar
Shrimp	Fit Factor
White fish	Julian's Bakery Paleo Bars
Pork Loin	Atkins Lift Protein Bar
Salmon	Atkins Lift Bars
	ANSI Gourmet Cheesecake Bars

APPROVED WHEY PROTEIN

Quest

ISO 100

Pure Protein

Designer Whey

PE Science

Garden of Life

Bownar

Paleo Protein

About Time

Optimum Nutrition Gold Standard

Evolve

Olympian Labs Pea Protein

Health Warriors Superfood

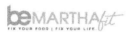

This plan is owned by #beMarthaFit and is not to be copied, recreated, or reproduced in any way. If you do not follow this plan 100 percent, you will not achieve your desired results. One hundred percent effort and consistency are the keys to this plan.

High-Fat 1,600-Calorie Plan

Average Calories: 1,600 | Protein: 121 | Fat: 100 | Carbs: 82

Breakfast Options: Pick one and alternate:

1. Egg Sandwich: 2 plant power cauliflower bread thins (link at bottom) plus 1 egg and 1 slice of cheese.
2. 3 full egg with 2 pieces of nitrate free turkey bacon and 1 cup of spinach/greens. May make into an omelet.
3. Low Carb French Toast Egg Puffs, recipe sent. Eat 2
4. Low carb waffle/pancake: combine 2 eggs, 1 scoop protein and ¼ tsp. baking powder and any spices you would like. Changing protein powders gives lots of variety. Blend and make into a waffle or pancakes. With 1 TBS of nut butter. May top with sugar free syrup and spray butter. Top with ½ cup of berries. These toast well so you can make a big batch and throw in the toaster the morning of.
5. Keto Instant Hot Cereal (link at bottom) 1.5 servings. May top with berries.

Morning Snack Options: Pick one and alternate:

1. Pecan Cheesecake Muffins, recipe provided. Eat plus 1 cheese stick
2. Oikos black label Greek yogurt place 1 ounce of walnuts.
3. Approved Bar. Please see guideline sheet below for list of approved options.

Lunch Guidelines:

5 ounces protein and 1 cup of veggies. Note: You do not have to use lean meat only. You can use salmon and steak here. No corn, sweet peas or carrots. Please see guideline sheet below for list of approved options

You may make this a salad. Use 2 cups of spinach and filler veggies with your protein. Use Bolthouse or Walden Farms dressing. Pay attention to serving size on label of dressing

Added fat: Pick one: ½ of medium avocado, 1 ounce of mozzarella, 1 ounce of 70% or above dark chocolate, 1 egg, ½ ounce of walnuts, 10 almonds or 1 ounce of chia seeds.

Afternoon Snack Options: Pick one and alternate:

1. Caprese Salad: 1 cup grape tomatoes, 4 ounces mozzarella and 1TBS of balsamic vinegar.
2. Chef Casey's deviled eggs, recipe sent. Plus 1 cheese stick.
3. Celery and 2 TBS of nut butter

Dinner Guidelines:

1. 5 ounces protein and 1 cup of veggies. Please see guideline sheet below for list of approved options
2. **Added fat:** Pick one: ½ of medium avocado, 1 ounce of mozzarella, 1 ounce of 70% or above dark chocolate, 1 egg, ½ ounce of walnuts, 10 almonds or 1 ounce of chia seeds.

Evening Snack Option:

1. Halo Top Ice Cream: 1 serving
2. Protein shake
3. Chef Casey's cake in a mug, recipe provided.
4. Oikos black label Greek yogurt

Plantpower Bread Thins. YOU CAN ALSO GET THESE AT WEGMAN'S!
https://www.outeraislegourmet.com/?gclid=EAIaIQobChMI8tX0yNCl4wIVz-FYNCh08EQSxEAAYASAAEgISbvD_BwE

Instant Keto Cereal:
https://www.amazon.com/gp/product/B07JP79VQZ/ref=ppx_yo_dt_b_asin_title_o08_s00?ie=UTF8&psc=1

APPROVED LEAN PROTEINS

Chicken breast	Shrimp
Lean ground turkey	White fish
Lean ground beef	Pork Loin
Flank steak	Salmon

APPROVED PROTEIN BARS

Atkins Snack Bar
Quest Hero Bars
No Cow
Quest Beyond Cereal Bar
Julians Bakery Paleo Bars
Atkins Lift Protein Bar
Atkins Lift Bars
ANSI Gourmet Cheesecake Bars

APPROVED WHEY PROTEIN

Quest
ISO 100
Pure Protein
Designer Whey
PE Science
Garden of Life
Bownar
Paleo Protein
About Time
Optimum Nutrition Gold Standard
Evolve
Olympian Labs Pea Protein
Health Warriors Superfood

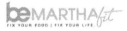

This plan is owned by #beMarthaFit and is not to be copied, recreated, or reproduced in any way. If you do not follow this plan 100 percent, you will not achieve your desired results. One hundred percent effort and consistency are the keys to this plan.

High-Fat 1,800-Calorie Plan

Average Calories: 1,828 | Protein: 185 | Fat: 97 | Carbs: 72

Breakfast Options: Pick one and alternate:

1. Egg Sandwich: 2 plant power cauliflower bread thins (link at bottom) plus 1 egg and 1 slice of cheese.
2. 3 full egg with 2 pieces of nitrate free turkey bacon and 1 cup of spinach/greens. May make into an omelet.
3. Chocolate Protein Donut, recipe provided. Eat 4
4. Low carb waffle/pancake: combine 2 eggs, 1 scoop protein and ¼ tsp. baking powder and any spices you would like. Changing protein powders gives lots of variety. Plus 1 TBS of peanut butter. Blend and make into a waffle or pancakes. May also top with spray butter or sugar free syrup or heavy whipped topping and ½ cup of berries. These toast well so you can make a big batch and throw in the toaster the morning of.
5. Quick Crunch "Cereal", recipe provided. Eat 1 serving.

Morning Snack Options: Pick one and alternate:

1. Low Carb Macadamia Nut Granola, recipe sent. Eat 1 serving
2. Pumpkin Maple Flaxseed Muffins, recipe sent. Eat 2
3. Oikos black label Greek yogurt plus ¼ cup of pecans.
4. Celery and 2.5 TBS of nut butter.

Lunch Guidelines:

7 ounces protein and 2 cups of veggies. Note: You do not have to use lean meat only. You can use salmon and steak here. No corn, sweet peas or carrots. Please see guideline sheet below for list of approved options

You may make this a salad. Use 2 cups of spinach and filler veggies with your protein. Use Bolthouse or Walden Farms dressing. Pay attention to serving size on label of dressing.

Added fat: Pick one: ½ of medium avocado, 1 ounce of mozzarella, 1 ounce of 70% or above dark chocolate, 1 egg, ½ ounce of walnuts, 10 almonds or 1 ounce of chia seeds.

Afternoon Snack Options: Pick one and alternate:

1. Chef Casey's Cheesy Chicken Quesadilla, recipe sent. Plus 10 plain almonds.
2. Chef Casey's Deviled Eggs, recipe sent. Eat 4 plus 2 cheese sticks OR 1 TBS of nut butter.
3. Approved protein bar. Plus 1 cheese stick OR 10 plain almonds. Please see guideline sheet below for list of approved options

Dinner Guidelines:

7 ounces protein and 2 cups of veggies. Please see guideline sheet below for list of approved options.

Added fat: Pick one: ½ of medium avocado, 1 ounce of mozzarella, 1 ounce of 70% or above dark chocolate, 1 egg, ½ ounce of walnuts, 10 almonds or 1 ounce of chia seeds.

Evening Snack Option:

1. Halo Top Ice Cream: 1.5 servings
2. Protein shake
3. Chef Casey's Cake in Mug, recipe provided.
4. 4 ounces of lunch meat OR 2 ounces of lunch meat and 1 ounce of cheese. Can wrap it around the cheese

Plantpower Bread Thins. YOU CAN ALSO GET THESE AT WEGMAN'S! https://www.outeraislegourmet.com/?gclid=EAIaIQobChMI8tX0yNCl4wIVz-FYNCh08EQSxEAAYASAAEgISbvD_BwE

Instant Keto Cereal: https://www.amazon.com/gp/product/B07JP79VQZ/ref=ppx_yo_dt_b_asin_title_o08_s00?ie=UTF8&psc=1

APPROVED LEAN PROTEINS

Chicken breast
Lean ground turkey
Lean ground beef
Flank steak
Shrimp
White fish
Pork Loin
Salmon

APPROVED PROTEIN BARS

Atkins Snack Bar
Quest Hero Bars
No Cow
Quest Beyond Cereal Bar
Julians Bakery Paleo Bars
Atkins Lift Protein Bar
Atkins Lift Bars
ANSI Gourmet Cheesecake Bars

APPROVED WHEY PROTEIN

Quest
ISO 100
Pure Protein
Designer Whey
PE Science
Garden of Life
Bownar
Paleo Protein
About Time
Optimum Nutrition Gold Standard
Evolve
Olympian Labs Pea Protein
Health Warriors Superfood

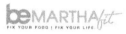

This plan is owned by #beMarthaFit and is not to be copied, recreated, or reproduced in any way. If you do not follow this plan 100 percent, you will not achieve your desired results. One hundred percent effort and consistency are the keys to this plan.

Carb Cycling Meal Plan

Average Calories: 1,400 High/1,200–1,300 Low

Note: you can use this plan with any type of carb cycling. Example, 2 days high, 1 day low. Or 2 days high, 5 days low.

Breakfast Options: High Day Pick one:

1. 1/2 cup of oats and 2x the water, microwaved. Add in 1 scoop of whey protein. Top with either: ½ cup of berries or cherries or ½ banana
2. French Toast, recipe provided. Eat 1.5 servings. May top with spray butter and sugar free jelly.

Low Day Pick one:

1. Egg Quiche Muffins, recipe provided. Eat 3
2. Low Carb Pancake/Waffle, recipe provided. Plus 2 pieces of nitrate free turkey bacon
   Recipe: Blend together 2 large eggs, 1 scoop of protein powder, ¼ tsp of baking powder and any spices you like (i.e. cinnamon). Make into pancakes or waffles. Top with sugar-free syrup and also have ½ cup of berries.

Morning Snack Options: Pick one and alternate:

High Day

Lemon Muffins, recipe provided. Eat 3

Low Day

2 ounces of fattier beef or salmon and 2 cups of greens or Cheesy Biscuit, recipe provided. Eat 1

Lunch Guidelines:

4 ounces lean protein, 1 cup of veggies and ½ cup complex carb. Carb only on high days. Increase veggies to 1.5 cup on low day. Please see guideline sheet below for list of approved options

Afternoon Snack Options:

High Day

Pumpkin Muffin, recipe provided. Eat 2 or Approved protein bar
Please see guideline sheet below for list of approved options

Low Day

Protein shake and 1 TBS of Natural Peanut Butter

Dinner Guidelines:

4 ounces lean protein and 2 cups of veggies. ½ cup of complex carb
on high day and on low day increase veggies to 1.5 cups. Please see
guideline sheet below for list of approved options

Evening Snack Option:

Halo Top or Enlightened Ice Cream 1.5 servings
Protein shake

APPROVED LEAN PROTEINS

Chicken breast
Lean ground turkey
Lean ground beef
Flank steak 2x a week
Salmon 2x a week
Shrimp
White fish
Pork Loin

APPROVED PROTEIN BARS

BSN Crisp
Quest
No Cow
Grenade
Combat
Kirkland
Oh Yeah One
Pure Protein
Think Thin High Protein
Fit Factor

APPROVED WHEY PROTEIN

Quest

ISO 100

Pure Protein

Designer Whey

PE Science

Garden of Life

Bownar

Paleo Protein

About Time

Evolve

Olympian Labs Pea Protein

Health Warriors Superfood

APPROVED COMPLEX CARBS

Brown rice

Sweet potatoes

Couscous

Quinoa

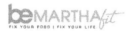

This plan is owned by #beMarthaFit and is not to be copied, recreated, or reproduced in any way. If you do not follow this plan 100 percent, you will not achieve your desired results. One hundred percent effort and consistency are the keys to this plan.

Mocktails

PALOMA MOCKTAIL

- Unsweetened Grapefruit Juice
- Sparkling, Seltzer or Soda Water (plain or flavored)
- 1 Limes
- 1 Grapefruit
- Truvia or Stevia (optional)

In a highball glass combine grapefruit juice, plain or flavored seltzer water, fresh squeezed lime juice. Stir, add ice and garnish with grapefruit slice.

MARGARITA MOCKTAIL

- Lime
- No Salt Substitute or Pink Himalayan Salt
- Truvia or Stevia
- Lemon Lime BCAA
- Water or Sparkling Water

Run a lime wedge around the rim of your margarita glass and lightly coat with Truvia, Stevia, No Salt Substitute or Pink Himalayan salt. In a shaker combine ice, water, Lemon Lime BCAAs and shake. Pour mixture into rimmed glass and garnish with fresh lime. Serve on the rocks or frozen.

TIP: If you're going out to a restaurant, bring BCAA's with you. Order a glass of ice water or soda water with a lime wedge & assemble yourself at the table.

MOJITO MOCKTAIL

- Fresh Mint Leaves or Mint Essential Oils
- Lime
- Truvia or Stevia
- Sparkling, Seltzer or Soda water (any flavor)

In a Collins glass, muddle fresh mint leaves, lime and 1 packet of Truvia in a glass. Pour in your choice of seltzer water. Gently stir and pour over ice. Garnish with a lime wedge and mint.

PIÑA COLADA MOCKTAIL

- Piña Colada BANG Drink
- Sugar Free Coconut Water
- Fresh Frozen Pineapple Chunks
- Sugar Free Whipped Topping
- Pineapple
- Fresh Cherries

In a blender combine a piña colada flavored Bang drink, coconut water, frozen pineapple, and ice. Pour mixture into a poco grande glass and top with sugar free whipped topping, a fresh cherry and a pineapple slice.

WILD BERRY LEMONADE MOCKTAIL

- Fresh Mixed Berries of your choice
- Lemon
- Truvia or Stevia
- Lemon Seltzer Water
- Lemon BCAAs (optional)

In a mason jar or Collins glass muddle berries and fresh lemon juice, and a Truvia packet. Pour in your favorite lemon-flavored seltzer water. Stir and add crushed ice. (serve on the rocks or frozen) Garnish with a lemon wedge and berries.

POMEGRANATE MOCKTAIL

- Sparkling, Seltzer or Soda Water (Any flavor)
- POM Juice
- Fresh Pomegranate
- Lime
- Truvia or Stevia
- No Salt Substitute

In a highball glass combine sparkling water, POM, fresh squeezed lime juice and pomegranate. Stir, add ice and garnish with a lime wedge.

SANGRIA MOCKTAIL

- Spindrift Raspberry-Lime Seltzer (or any flavored seltzer water of your choice)
- Unsweetened Orange Juice
- POM
- Fresh squeezed Lemon & Lime Juice
- Orange
- Berry BCAAs (optional)

In a large pitcher combine the above ingredients. Stir, add chunks of mixed fruit and ice. Serve in a long stem glass and garnish with a lime wedge.

BLOODY MARY MOCKTAIL

- Low Sodium Tomato Juice
- Low Sodium Seafood Seasoning
- Coconut Aminos (or Liquid Aminos)
- Lime
- Horseradish
- Hot Sauce (optional)

Run a lime wedge along the rim of a highball glass and coat with low sodium seafood seasoning. Combine low sodium tomato juice, juice from 1 lime, and a dash of coconut aminos. Add celery salt, and horseradish. Stir, add ice and garnish with a celery stalk and a lime wedge.

MOSCOW MULE MOCKTAIL

- Diet Ginger-ale or Sugar Free Ginger Beer
- Plain Sparkling Water
- Lime
- Fresh Ginger or Ginger Essential Oil (optional)

In a copper mug combine Sparkling water, Diet Ginger-ale, fresh squeezed lime juice and a few slices of fresh ginger. Stir, add crushed ice and garnish with a lime wheel and mint

STRAWBERRY DAIQUIRI MOCKTAIL

- Frozen Strawberries
- Water or flavored seltzer water
- Lime
- Sugar Free Whipped Topping

In a blender combine frozen strawberries, water, and lime juice. Pour mixture into a cocktail glass and garnish with sugar free whipped topping and a strawberry.

Monthly Goals

Date:

Addition: What are you going to add in the next 30 days to help you achieve your goal?

Elimination: What are you going to eliminate this month? Remember this cannot be focused on pounds lost on the scale. Examples: Are you willing to commit to no alcohol for the next 30 days? Are you willing to commit to no junk food for the next 30 days? Are you willing to commit to no soda for the next 30 days?

Remember to check in with yourself on Wednesday. How are you doing? Anything you need to add or eliminate to help you reach your goals? Keep goals simple. Do not over-complicate them.

Measurement (Body) Guide

How Often Should I Weigh Myself? It is recommended that you pick one day each week that you weigh yourself on. For example, I weigh myself every Monday. There is no need to weigh yourself daily. If you are following a weight loss meal plan 100 percent, you can expect to lose 1–3 pounds every 7–10 days.

What about Progress Pictures? It is recommended that you pick one day a month to take progress pictures of yourself. Trust me, fast forward three months from now, and you'll be glad you did so you can see all of the progress you've made. Take full-length body shots in form-fitting clothing (athletic shorts and shirt are fine). If you can, try to stand in the same spot every time. Take a photo from the front, side, and back of your body. Get someone else to take the photos if you are comfortable. You can share these images or just keep them in an album on your mobile device to help track your own progress.

> **Before and After Progress Pictures.** This is typically a comparison of your progress after three or more months. You will want to position your most recent image on the right and the older picture on the left. Keep it simple. You need only two images for your before and after collage.

How to take Body Measurements. The scale is not the end all, be all. Some prefer to take measurements and never weigh themselves at all. It is recommended that you take measurements at the start of your meal plan then continue to take and record your measurements monthly. All you'll need to measure your progress is a soft, flexible measuring tape. Be sure to measure around your chest, right across the nipple line, and measure your waist across your belly button. Measure each upper arm around the biggest part. Measure your hips by placing the tape measure around the widest part of your hips. Lastly, you'll want to measure each thigh around the biggest part as well. Remember you only need to do this every four weeks to track your progress. If you're following your meal plan, consistently eating at a healthy caloric deficit that's right for you, you will lose weight. Stay focused.

Progress Chart Example

Start date:
Weight:

Week 1
Weight:

Week 2
Weight:

Week 3
Weight:

Week 4
Weight:

Month 1:
Weight:
Total pounds lost:
Non-scale victories:

Note: Continue this format for one month at a time.

Recipes—Breakfast

Cinnamon Roll Coffee Cake

Nutrition Facts:

106 Calories | 12g Protein | 9 g Carbs | 2 g Fat
Prep Time: 20 mins
Cooking Time: 25 mins
Servings: 8

Ingredients:

- 2 scoops vanilla protein powder
- 1 cup Kodiak Buttermilk Pancake Mix
- ⅔ cup of nonfat yogurt
- 2 large eggs
- ¼ cup sweetener (optional)
- 1 tsp of vanilla
- 1 TBS sugar free maple syrup
- Filling: 2 tbs swerve brown sugar and 1.5 tbs cinnamon
- Icing: 1 tbs vanilla protein powder, 1tbs whipped cream cheese, 1.5 cashew milk and 1 tbs swerve confectioners sugar

Directions:

1. In a large mixing bowl combine protein powder, pancake mix, sweetener and blend. Add two eggs and slowly add yogurt till you have dough consistency. A little less than ⅔ cup. Mix dough well with a spoon and knead.
2. On a baking sheet place parchment paper and spray lightly with cooking spray. Roll out dough or use hands to flatten and shape dough into a rectangle or oval (about 10-12 inches width and length). Refrigerate 20 mins. Preheat the oven to 375 when dough goes into the fridge.

3. Prepare filling in a small dish. When dough comes out of the fridge drizzle with the sugar free maple syrup over dough and sprinkle filling. Roll the dough up tight like a tube and bake 20-25 mins. Doubt should look done and slightly golden. Remove from the oven.

4. Prepare the icing and drizzle over top of the coffee cake. Let cool 5-10 mins and then cut into 8 equal pieces.

Apple Fritters

Nutrition Facts:

95 Calories | 12g Protein | 8g Carbs | 1g Fat

Prep Time: 10 mins
Cooking Time: 15 mins
Servings: 9

Ingredients:

- ¾ cup buttermilk Kodiak power cake mix
- 2 scoops of vanilla protein powder
- 2 eggs
- ½ cup of nonfat Greek yogurt
- 2/4 cup swerve brown sugar
- 1 medium apple, cored, peeled and chopped
- 1 tsp vanilla
- 1 tsp cinnamon
- 2 tsp baking powder
- 2 Tbsp apple cider vinegar

Directions:

1. Preheat oven to 350 degrees
2. In a mixing bowl combine all dry ingredients and blend well.
3. Add in eggs and mix, then add in yogurt and continue to mix. Batter will be dry. Once well blended add 1 Tbsp of vinegar at a time. The batter should be doughy and sticky. Stir in chopped apple.
4. On a well sprayed baking sheet drop 9 equal portions and bake 15-17 mins.
5. Note: Dough consistency will depend on the type of powder used. You may have to slowly add water to find doughy sticky consistency.
6. Macros based on 1 fritter

Apple Turkey Muffins

Nutrition Facts:

144 Calories | 17g Protein | 7g Carbs | 6g Fat

Prep Time: 10 mins
Cooking Time: 25 mins
Servings: 6

Ingredients:

- Dash of black pepper
- ¼ tsp ground nutmeg
- ¾ tsp cinnamon
- ¼ cup chopped onions
- ½ cup unsweetened applesauce
- 4 Tbsp 100% liquid egg whites
- ½ cup uncooked old fashioned oats
- 16 ounces 93% fat free ground turkey

Directions:

1. Preheat oven to 350 degrees
2. Finely chop onions in a food processor. Combine all ingredients in a large bowl. Mix well.
3. Spray a muffin tin with cooking spray. Evenly divide the turkey mixture into muffin tin.
4. Bake for 25 minutes and serve.

Banana Bread Protein Smoothie

Nutrition Facts:

412 Calories | 34.5g Protein | 40.8g Carbs | 13.1g Fat

Prep Time: 2 mins
Cooking Time: None
Servings: 1

Ingredients:

- ½ cup of low-fat cottage cheese
- ½ cup of vanilla almond milk
- ½ medium banana (frozen or fresh)
- 1 scoop of vanilla protein powder
- 2 Tbsp chopped walnuts
- ½ tsp vanilla extract
- 1 tsp cinnamon
- ½ tsp nutmeg

Directions:

Blend all the ingredients together until smooth. Enjoy!

Apple Protein Pancake

Nutrition Facts:

296 Calories | 34g Protein | 27g Carbs | 6g Fat

Prep Time: 10 mins
Cooking Time: 10 mins
Servings: 1

Ingredients:

- 1 egg
- 2 egg whites
- 3 Tbsp unsweetened almond milk
- 1 scoop protein powder
- 1 medium apple cored and diced
- 1 tsp vanilla extract
- 1 tsp or more cinnamon
- ¼ tsp baking powder
- 1 tsp or to taste sweetener of choice
- 1 Tbsp sugar free maple syrup (optional and not included in macros)

Directions:

1. In a well-sprayed frying pan add diced apples, cinnamon, sweetener and optional maple syrup to taste. Cook until apples are soft and browned. Set aside.
2. In a small mixing bowl beat egg and egg whites and remaining ingredients until smooth batter. This will take a few minutes as the protein powder breaks down.
3. Pour into a heated skillet. Add apples to batter and cook as you would a regular pancake.
4. You can substitute apples for blueberries!

Lunch and Dinner

Asian Crack Slaw

Nutrition Facts:

270 Calories | 30g Protein | 12g Carbs | 11g Fat

Prep Time: 5
Cooking Time: 20
Servings: 4

Ingredients:

- 1 ¼ lb lean 93/7 ground turkey
- 1 Tbsp sriracha
- 2 cloves of garlic
- 1 tsp rice vinegar
- 1 Tbsp sesame seed oil
- ¼ tsp black pepper
- 2 Tbsp liquid aminos
- ½ tsp pink himalayan sea salt
- 1 tsp sesame seeds
- 6 cups coleslaw salad mix
- 1 stalk green onion

Directions:

1. Heat sesame oil in a large pan. Add garlic and cook until fragrant. Add ground turkey and cook until browned.
2. Weigh ground turkey and divide into containers if meal prepping or on a plate for dinner according to your meat ounces on your plan.
3. Add slaw, sriracha, liquid aminos and vinegar to the pan and cook for 5 minutes or until cabbage/salad mix is wilted.
4. Season with salt, pepper and sesame seeds. Garnish with green onion.
5. Makes 4 servings. Macros based on 4oz portions of meat.

Creamy Chicken Jalapeno Enchiladas

Nutrition Facts:

209 Calories | 26g Protein | 11g Carbs | 8g Fat

Prep Time: 30 mins
Cooking Time: 30 mins
Servings: 8

Ingredients:

- 1.5 lbs. cooked and shredded boneless skinless chicken breast (suggested cooking method is crockpot on high 4 hours with seasonings and 2 Tbsp chicken broth)
- 1 Tbsp Tone's Cilantro lime seasoning or any fiesta blend low sodium seasoning
- 1 tsp cumin
- 1 Tbsp garlic powder
- 1 Tbsp onion powder
- 1 tsp chili powder
- 1 tsp paprika
- 2-3 jalapenos deveined, seeded and diced (if you want hot leave in veins) plus one sliced for garnish
- ½ onion diced
- Sauce: 2 small cans low sodium diced green chilis and 1 container of fresh salsa or pico de gallo
- 2 whole wheat lavash bread
- 8 ounces whipped cream cheese (Look for Greek yogurt whipped cream cheese if you can… Kroger)
- ⅓ cup reduced fat shredded cheese

Directions:

1. Season and prepare chicken as you wish using suggested seasonings
2. In a food processor or blender combine green chilis, fresh salsa and suggested seasoning and puree (enchilada sauce).

3. When chicken is cooked and shredded start this next step. In a well sprayed frying pan saute diced jalapenos and onion about 7 minutes on medium heat. Add chicken and mix. Next add cream cheese and a Tbsp or two of your enchilada sauce. Continue to stir until cream cheese is melted through. Turn off heat.

4. In a well sprayed 9x13 baking dish spread a small amount of sauce on the bottom. Lay one lavash sheet down and spread half of the chicken mixture then half of the sauce. Repeat this step. Finish with diced jalapenos and shredded cheese.

5. Bake at 350 degrees for 30-40 minutes.

6. Cut into 8 equal portions. Macros based on 1 portion.

Fried Chicken Fingers

Nutrition Facts:

159 Calories |24 g Protein | 15g Carbs | 2g Fat

Prep Time: 10 mins
Cooking Time: 15 mins
Servings: 4

Ingredients:

- 1 lb. boneless skinless chicken breast cut into strips or bite size pieces
- 2.5 cups bran flakes, measure out then crush flakes (use corn flakes if gluten free)
- 1 Tbsp Parmesan cheese
- 1 tsp oregano, paprika, garlic powder and any other low sodium seasoning, Make it yours add your own twist!
- 2 egg whites

Directions:

1. Preheat oven to 400 degrees
2. Dip chicken pieces into egg whites and then into bran crumbs. Place on a well sprayed baking sheet or air fryer basket.
3. Once all chicken is dipped and on the pan, coat chicken with cooking spray.
4. Bake or air fry for 15-18 minutes.
5. Macros are based on 4 ounce portions.

Loaded Baked Potato Soup

Nutrition Facts:

177 Calories | 19g Protein | 10g Carbs | 7g Fat

Prep Time: 10
Cooking Time: 30 mins
Servings: 5

Ingredients:

- 1 medium russet potato (10-15 ounces precooked) skinned and cut into small cubes
- ½ cup diced onion
- 1 Tbsp crushed garlic
- ½ tsp xanthan gum (this can be skipped but helps thicken the soup)
- 4 cups of no salt added chicken broth
- 2 scoops unflavored protein powder
- 2 stalks green onion, chopped
- 3 slices nitrate free turkey bacon, cooked and crumbled
- black pepper to taste
- ½ tsp pink Himalayan salt
- 12 oz frozen cauliflower rice
- ¾ cup shredded low-fat cheddar cheese

Directions:

1. In 4 qt. pot on medium heat spray bottom and saute onions and garlic 4 minutes and then add xanthan gum. Stir and let cook for one more minute. Add diced potatoes, crumbled bacon and 2 cups of broth. Turn to low and let simmer for 30 minutes.

2. In a blender, blend 2 cups chicken broth with 2 scoops unflavored protein powder until well blended.

3. When potatoes are tender add cauliflower rice and blended broth protein powder to the pot. Stir in well and let simmer on low for 10 more minutes.

4. Add cheese and green onions and stir until the cheese is well blended. Salt and pepper to taste.

5. Macros based on 5 1 cup portions of soup.

Shrimp Gumbo

Nutrition Facts:

164 Calories | 28g Protein | 21g Carbs | 2g Fat

Prep Time: 10
Cooking Time: 4-6 hours
Servings: 10

Ingredients:

- 2 lbs peeled and tails off medium size cooked shrimp
- 14.5 oz. no salt added diced tomatoes
- 1 green bell pepper
- 1 cup yellow onion, diced
- 4 stalks celery, chopped
- 15 oz can kidney beans
- ½ cup uncooked rice
- 6 cups no salt added chicken broth
- 2 Tbsp crushed garlic
- 1 Tbsp garlic powder
- 1 Tbsp minced onion
- 2 tsp liquid smoke
- 2 tsp smoked paprika
- 2 bay leaves
- ½-1 tsp cayenne pepper (optional)
- 1 tsp oregano
- 1 tsp thyme
- 1 tsp black pepper
- 1 tsp pink himalayan salt

Directions:

1. Turn the crockpot on low and add all ingredients except rice and shrimp. Let simmer for 5 to 6 hours.
2. Add rice and continue to cook for 45 minutes.
3. Add shrimp and let simmer for 15 minutes more.
4. Macros based on 1 cup serving. Makes 10 servings.

Korean Beef Bowl

Nutrition Facts:

178 Calories | 23g Protein | 3g Carbs | 9g Fat

Prep Time: 15minutes
Cooking Time: 15 minutes
Servings: 8

Ingredients:

- 2 lbs lean ground beef (93% or 96%)
- 1 tbsp low sodium Asian seasoning(optional)
- 1 tbsp minced onion
- 1 tbsp garlic powder
- 1 tsp ginger powder
- Sauce: 1/3 cup coconut amino acids, 2 tsp sweet or spicy chili garlic sauce, 1 tsp sesame oil or chili pepper oil, 2 tbsp crushed garlic, 1 tsp crushed ginger, 1 tbsp Swerve brown sugar (optional)
- A variety of raw veggies diced—bell peppers (use all the colors), mushrooms, onion, broccoli, cucumbers—whatever your family likes.

Directions:

1. In a large well sprayed medium heat skillet brown meat adding garlic powder, minced onion, ginger powder, and low sodium Asian seasoning.
2. Combine sauce ingredients and whisk. Add to cooked meat and stir. Low heat 2 or 3 minutes.
3. Suggested way to serve: In a bowl combine your portion of jasmine rice or cauliflower rice, add meat portion and desired veggies of choice. Drizzle with your favorite low sodium sweet or spicy Asian sauce and enjoy!

Macros based on 4 oz meat and sauce portions only.

#beMarthaFit Pizza

Nutrition Facts Per Serving

226 Calories | 23g Protein | 21g Carbs | 5g FatPrep Time: 10 minutes
Cooking Time: 18 minutes
Servings: 4

Ingredients:

- 1 1/4 cups Kodiak buttermilk pancake mix
- 2 scoops unflavored protein powder
- 1 cup + 2 tbsp hot water (add slowly you do not want this dough to be wet)
- Optional 1 tbsp low sodium Italian seasoning or garlic powder
- 1/2 cup low sodium pizza, spaghetti, marinara or tomato sauce
- 3/4 cup skim mozzarella cheese
- Olive oil cooking spray

Directions:

1. Preheat oven to 400 degrees
2. In a large mixing bowl combine pancake mix, protein powder and seasoning. Slowly add water while spoon mixing. Spray mixture for 3 seconds with olive oil cooking spray (this will help with forming dough). When liquid is absorbed begin hand mixing. Dough should just slightly stick to your hands.
3. Place parchment paper on baking sheet and begin to roll out or hand flatten dough. Shape into about a 12" circle. Spray top of dough with olive oil cooking spray and bake about 8 mins. Dough can be as thick or thin as you like. My family likes it thin.
4. Remove pizza dough from oven and spread 1/2 cup low sodium pizza, marinara, spaghetti or tomato sauce over top. Season as you would like. Sprinkle 3/4 cup skim mozzarella cheese and bake 8-10 mins more or until desired doneness.Macros based on 1/4 of cheese pizza. Toppings not included in listed macros.

Pizza is macro balanced as is. 3oz of protein can be added as well as veggies of any sort if desired .

Amazing Beef

Nutrition Facts Per Serving

162 Calories | 23g Protein | 0g Carbs | 6g Fat

Prep Time: 1 minute
Cooking Time: 4-6 Hours
Servings: 8

Ingredients:

- 2lb Chuck tender roast or flank steak
- 1 16 oz jar peperoncini (sliced or whole)
- 1 tbsp garlic powder

Directions:

1. In crock pot set heat to low. Add beef and half jar of pepperoncini juice and half the pepperoncini and garlic powder
2. Cook 4 to 6 hours until beef falls apart
3. Eat on a 647 hoagie style bun or over rice or shredded cabbage
4. Be sure to drizzle juice over beef and just a dash of parmesan cheese

Macros based on 4 oz portion of beef

Snacks

Peanut Butter Protein Bombs

Nutrition Facts Per Serving

33 Calories |5g Protein | 1g Carbs | 1g Fat

Prep time: 5 minutes
Cooking time: 0
Servings: 1

Ingredients:

- 1 scoop vanilla protein powder
- 4 tbsp peanut butter powder
- 1 tsp or more Swerve confectioners sugar (to your desired sweetness)
- 2 tbsp unsweetened applesauce
- 4 tbsp unsweetened cashew or almond milk

Directions:

1. In a small bowl combine all dry ingredients and blend.
2. Add 2 tbs applesauce and then add 1 tbs milk at a time (slowly) mixing between each until a firm dough forms.
3. Shape into 6 balls and put in freezer for 30 mins!

Macros based on 1 bal

Banana Bread Pudding

Nutrition Facts Per Serving

158 Calories | 15g Protein | 12g Carbs | 6g Fat

Ingredients:

- Prep Time: 5 minutes
- Cooking Time: 50 minutes
- Servings: 8
- 2 very ripe bananas
- 2 large eggs
- 1 cup nonfat Greek yogurt
- 1 tsp vanilla
- 3 scoops protein powder
- 8 tbs almond flour
- 3/4 cup Swerve brown sugar
- 1 tsp baking powder
- 1 tsp baking soda
- 2 servings Lily's baking chips

Directions:

1. In a mixing bowl mash two ripe bananas until almost runny, then add remaining wet ingredients and swerve brown sugar.
2. Mix until well blended.
3. Add dry ingredients one at a time and mix until well blended then add chocolate chips.
4. Pour batter into a well sprayed bread pan.
5. Bake at 350 degrees for 45-50 mins

Macros based on 1 slice

Pecan White Chocolate Chip Cookies

Nutrition Facts Per Serving

68 Calories | 5g Protein | 2g Carbs | 5g Fat

Prep Time: 5 minutes
Cooking Time: 15 minutes
Servings: 12

Ingredients:

- 12 tbs Pecan Flour
- 2 scoops vanilla protein powder (I use Iconic)
- 1 tsp baking powder
- 3-4 tbsp brown sugar swerve
- 1 tsp maple or vanilla extract
- 1 serving choc zero white chocolate chips or Lily's baking chips
- 2 egg whites
- 1 whole egg
- 1/2 cup unsweetened apple sauce OR 1/2 cup pumpkin puree

Directions:

1. Preheat the oven to 350.Combine all dry ingredients and mix.
2. Add wet ingredients and mix until well blended.
3. Drop 12 even size spoonfuls onto a well sprayed cookie sheet.
4. Bake at 350 degrees for 15 mins.

Macros based on 1 cookie

Sweet Potato Protein Brownies

Nutrition Facts Per Serving

98 Calories | 8g Protein | 6g Carbs | 4g Fat

Prep Time: 10 minutes
Cooking Time: 20 minutes
Servings: 9

Ingredients:

- 1 cup mashed sweet potato
- 1/4 cup all natural nut butter
- 2 scoops protein powder vanilla
- chocolate or peanut butter
- 2 egg whites
- 4 tbsp unsweetened cocoa powder
- 1 tsp or to taste sweetener
- 1 tsp baking powder
- 1/8 cup sugar free maple syrup
- 7 grams milk or dark chocolate chips
- 2 oz Unsweetened Almond milk (use 4 oz if not using espresso)
- 2 oz Espresso (optional)

Directions:

1. Combine in a bowl mashed sweet potatoes and peanut butter, mix. Add egg whites and protein powder, mix. Add almond milk (espresso), cocoa powder, baking powder, sweetener, mix

2. In a well sprayed 8x8 baking dish spread out batter and sprinkle chocolate chips evenly over top.

3. Bake at 350 for 15-20 mins

4. Cut into 9 even squares.

Macros based on 1 square. Store in refrigerator

Banana Bombs

Nutrition Facts Per Serving

220 Calories | 24g Protein | 21g Carbs | 4g Fat

Prep Time: 10 minutes
Cooking Time: 15-20 minutes
Servings: 5

Ingredients

- 4 to 5 scoops protein powder
- 2 large eggs
- 3 medium bananas mashed well
- 2 tbs chia seeds
- 1 tbs mini chocolate chips
- 1 tsp baking powder
- 1 tsp vanilla
- sweetener to taste (optional)

Directions

1. Mash banana then add protein, vanilla, and baking powder mix well. Stir in one egg at a time and mix until well blended. Fold in chia seed and mini chips.
2. On a well sprayed cookie sheet drop 5 even size portions.
3. Bake at 350 15-20 mins!
4. Macros based on one bomb!

Cheesy Garlic Bread

Nutrition Facts Per Serving

100 Calories | 12g Protein | 2g Carbs | 4g Fat

Prep Time: 10 minutes
Cooking Time: 20 minutes
Servings: 9

Ingredients

- ½ cup almond flour
- 3 scoops protein powder (Unflavored)
- 2 tsp baking powder
- 1 tbsp garlic powder
- 1 tbsp onion powder
- 1 tbsp OMS pizza or Weber garlic Parmesan (Optional depending if you want the flavor)
- 1 tsp rosemary or thyme (Optional depending on if you want this flavor)
- 1/3 cup low fat mozzarella cheese
- 4 egg whites
- 1tbs apple cider vinegar
- 4 tbsp unsweetened almond milk
- 2/3 cup nonfat yogurt

Directions

1. Mix dry ingredients together and then add wet ingredients. Mix shredded Cheese in last. Batter should be doughy and slightly sticky. Scoop evenly into 9 well sprayed muffin cups OR evenly scoop out 9 spoonful onto a well sprayed cookie shape. Dough should not be runny.
2. Bake at 325 for 18-22 mins
3. Makes 9 Biscuits or muffins
4. Macros based on 1 biscuit or muffin

Green Onion Deli Wrap

Nutrition Facts Per Serving

175 Calories | 23g Protein | 5g Carbs | 5g Fat

Prep Time: 5 minutes
Cooking Time: 0
Servings: 1

Ingredients

- 3 green onion stalks
- 2 wedges laughing cow cheese
- 3 oz Low sodium deli turkey

Directions

1. Spread cheese on deli turkey
2. Wrap turkey around a green onion stalk
3. Enjoy on its own or makes a great addition to a charcuterie spread!

CPSIA information can be obtained
at www.ICGtesting.com
Printed in the USA
BVHW030319020321
601385BV00005B/151